Immunology of the Gastrointestinal Tract

Volume II

Editors

Klara Miller

and

Stephen Nicklin

Department of Immunotoxicology
British Industrial Biological
Research Association
Carshalton, Surrey, England

CRC

CRC Press, Inc.
Boca Raton, Florida

Library of Congress Cataloging-in-Publication Data

Immunology of the gastrointestinal tract.

Includes bibliographies and index.
1. Gastrointestinal system--Diseases--Immunological aspects. 2. Antigens--Metabolism. 3. Immune response. 4. Food allergy. I. Miller, Klara. II. Nicklin, Stephen. [DNLM: 1. Gastrointestinal Diseases--immunology. 2. Gastrointestinal System--immunology. WI 100 I344]
RC817.I46 1987 616.3'3079 86-6072
ISBN 0-8493-4310-0 (Set)
ISBN 0-8493-4311-9 (v. 1)
ISBN 0-8493-4312-7 (v. 2)

Direct all inquiries to CRC Press, Inc., 2000 Corporate Blvd., N.W., Boca Raton, Florida, 33431.

International Standard Book Number 0-8493-4310-0 (Set)
International Standard Book Number 0-8493-4311-9 (Volume I)
International Standard Book Number 0-8493-4312-7 (Volume II)

Library of Congress Card Number 86-6072
Printed in the United States

FOREWORD

These volumes emphasize the importance of an intact gastrointestinal immune system in maintaining the health of the host. A detailed knowledge of the precise interactions that occur between ingested antigens and the intestinal immune system is clearly central to our understanding of the mechanisms governing such responses. With this view in mind we invited a number of internationally renowned scientists to write on their respective fields of interest. The extensive opening chapter by Professor Brandtzaeg traces the development and functions of local and systemic immune responses in man. Several chapters then explore whether these reactions are primary events, and hence can be regarded as basic causes of gastrointestinal syndromes.

Particular attention has been paid to recent research describing the unique properties of immunoglobulin A (IgA) and its rapid entry into the intestinal tract. Studies of responses to intestinal parasites are discussed in relation to the understanding they have given us of other intestinal responses within the gastrointestinal system including the initiation and regulation of IgE antibody formation and the origin and control of mucosal mast cells. Because of the current interest in food intolerance both the clinical symptoms and mechanisms involved in allergic and nonallergic responses to ingested materials are reviewed. The use of animal models in the study of immune responses and the development of more sophisticated laboratory techniques to unravel the complexities of these immune interactions and their regulation are also covered in some detail in the final section. We believe that these chapters will be of value to clinicians and immunologists alike.

The successful compilation of this book is due to the enthusiasm and care of the contributing authors and we are very grateful to them for providing such excellent chapters.

Klara Miller
Steve Nicklin

CONTRIBUTORS

E. M. Andrew
Division of Clinical Immunology
Kennedy Institute of Rheumatology
London, England

Peter Asquith
Consultant Physician and Gastroenterologist
Director of Metabolic Unit
East Birmingham Hospital
Birmingham, England

Kåre Baklien
Assistant Head Physician
Blood Bank and Department of Immunology
Ullevål Hospital
Oslo, Norway

Knut Bjerke
Research Fellow
Laboratory for Immunohistochemistry and Immunopathology
University of Oslo
The National Hospital, Rikshospitalet
Oslo, Norway

Per Brandtzaeg
Professor
Chief of Laboratory for Immunohistochemistry and Immunopathology
University of Oslo
The National Hospital, Rikshospitalet
Oslo, Norway

S. J. Challacombe
Department of Oral Immunology
Guys Hospital
United Medical and Dental Schools
London, England

R. K. Grencis
MRC Experimental Parasitology Group
Department of Zoology
University of Nottingham
Nottingham, England

Maurice H. Lessof
Professor
Department of Medicine
Guys Hospital
London, England

T. T. MacDonald
Department of Paediatric Gastroenterology
St. Bartholomew's Center for Clinical Research
London, England

Nigel Mike
Registrar
Metabolic and Clinical Investigation Unit
East Birmingham Hospital
Birmingham, England

Klara Miller
Head
Department of Immunotoxicology
British Industrial Biological Research Association
Carshalton, Surrey, England

Stephen Nicklin
Department of Immunotoxicology
British Industrial Biological Research Association
Carshalton, Surrey, England

Torleiv O. Rognum
Associate Professor
Institute of Forensic Medicine
University of Oslo
The National Hospital, Rikshospitalet
Oslo, Norway

Helge Scott
Assistant Physician
Department of Pathology
The National Hospital, Rikshospitalet
Oslo, Norway

Kolbjörn Valnes
Research Fellow
Laboratory for Immunohistochemistry and Immunopathology
Institute of Pathology
University of Oslo
The National Hospital, Rikshospitalet
Oslo, Norway

D. Wakelin
Professor
MRC Experimental Parasitology Group
Department of Zoology
University of Nottingham
Nottingham, England

TABLE OF CONTENTS

Volume I

Chapter 1
Nature and Properties of the Human Gastrointestinal Immune System 1
Per Brandtzaeg, Kåre Baklien, Knut Bjerke, Torleiv O. Rognum,
Helge Scott, and Kolbjörn Valnes

Chapter 2
Intestinal Uptake of Antigen: Immunological Consequences 87
Stephen Nicklin

Chapter 3
Mechanisms of Secretory IgA Responses 111
E. M. Andrew and T. T. MacDonald

Index 131

Volume II

Chapter 4
Immunological Responses to Intestinal Parasite Infection 1
D. Wakelin and R. K. Grencis

Chapter 5
Immune Responses in Chronic Gastrointestinal Diseases 25
Nigel Mike and Peter Asquith

Chapter 6
Diagnosis of Food Intolerance and Allergy...69
Maurice H. Lessof

Chapter 7
Intolerance to Food Colors and Other Additives..85
Klara Miller

Chapter 8
The Investigation of Secretory and Systemic Immune Responses to
Ingested Material in Animal Models 99
S. J. Challacombe

Index 127

Chapter 4

IMMUNOLOGICAL RESPONSES TO INTESTINAL PARASITE INFECTION

D. Wakelin and R. K. Grencis

TABLE OF CONTENTS

I. Introduction 2

II. Parasites and Immunity 2

III. Immune Effector Mechanisms 3

IV. Experimental Studies in Laboratory Models 4
A. Protozoa 4
1. Giardiasis 4
2. Coccidiosis 5
B. Platyhelminths 6
C. Nematoda 7

V. Experimental Studies in Domestic Animals 9
A. Coccidia 9
B. Nematoda 10

VI. Immune Responses in Man 11
A. Giardiasis 11
B. Intestinal Nematodes 11

VI. Immunological Consequences of Intestinal Infection 12
A. IgE 12
B. MMC 13
C. Eosinophils 14
D. Tolerance and Immunosuppression 15

VIII. Conclusions 16

Acknowledgments 16

References 16

I. INTRODUCTION

Gastrointestinal protozoa and helminths (worms) are probably the most common and most widespread of all parasitic organisms. Their prevalence and importance has prompted intensive studies of many aspects of their biology, with an increasing emphasis in the last 25 years on the immunological aspects of their host-parasite relationships. The goal of much of this research has been the application of immunological knowledge to improved diagnosis and prophylaxis, but there is no doubt that research interest has also been maintained by the many fundamental and intriguing questions which the continuing survival and success of these organisms pose.

The intestine has many mechanisms, both specific and nonspecific, to prevent colonization by infectious organisms and to reduce access of enterally presented antigens into the systemic circulation. Parasites have evolved to survive despite these mechanisms and release into the gut lumen or gut mucosa large amounts of antigenic material. How does the host succeed in controlling infection? What mechanisms can effectively deal with complex organisms that may be several millimeters or even several meters in length? How can these mechanisms be focused and expressed at sites of infection within the intestine? What systemic responses are there to enteral antigenic stimulation? It is well known that enteral stimulation can produce systemic tolerance (see below), and though this is clearly advantageous where food antigens are concerned, it could be disadvantageous in dealing with parasites. What relation does enteral recognition and response to antigen bear to systemic phenomena? Are mucosal defenses against parasites wholly independent from those operating against parenteral forms?

Studies of responses to intestinal parasites have thrown light on many of these questions and have illuminated a number of other immunological areas, e.g., the initiation and regulation of immunoglobulin E (IgE) antibody formation, the production and function of eosinophils, and the origin and control of mucosal mast cells. No attempt is made here to review comprehensively the very large literature dealing with immunological aspects of intestinal infection. This chapter is intended instead to introduce current ideas concerning the ability of hosts to control and overcome parasite invasion of the intestine and to serve as an overview of the insights that have been gained concerning both immune function in the intestine and the immunological consequences of intestinal infection.

II. PARASITES AND IMMUNITY

Intestinal parasites (defined here as protozoa and helminths) represent one of the most important groups of parasitic infections which afflict man and his domestic animals. Unlike other major parasites, such as malaria, trypanosomiasis, and schistosomiasis, they are infrequently associated with mortality in the infected population. They are, nevertheless, collectively responsible for an enormous degree of ill health and economic wastage. Characteristically, such infections are chronic in nature and produce low-grade, subclinical signs and symptoms. When infections are heavy, however, acute pathology, often inflammatory in origin, is induced. The prevalence of intestinal infections is, in part, a consequence of the evolutionary origins of parasitism. Entry into the host's body via the oral route and exit with fecal material are clearly the simplest and most straightforward pathways that a parasite species can use to establish infection and to release its reproductive stages. The persistence of such infections in human populations and in domestic animals is a consequence of socioeconomic and climatic conditions on the one hand, hence the prevalence of intestinal parasites in tropical/

subtropical regions, and of modern agricultural practices on the other hand, hence their prevalence in intensively reared and maintained livestock.

The chronicity of many intestinal infections raises the question of the effectiveness of immune responses against organisms parasitizing the gastrointestinal tract. While it was considered at one time that parasites were both poorly immunogenic and protected from effector mechanisms by virtue of their intestinal location, it is now well recognized that neither of these concepts is correct. Intestinal parasites are potent inducers of immune responses, and many species are dealt with very effectively by the responses which they evoke. Thus the phenomenon of ineffective protective immunity against other species, and particularly those associated with disease, introduces the possibilities that parasites may actively suppress or evade immune responses rather than fail to elicit them.

The study of immune responses to intestinal parasitic infections has been an active field of research for many years. From this work has come not only a greater insight into the ways in which hosts may protect themselves against infection but also a greater understanding of aspects of intestinal immunity and immunopathology which have much wider relevance. This review will therefore introduce both of these aspects. It will not, because of limitations on space, attempt to provide a comprehensive account of immunity to intestinal parasites, rather the emphasis will be upon work which the authors see as particularly significant or which provides growth points for future research.

III. IMMUNE EFFECTOR MECHANISMS

The general immunology of parasitic infections, including infections with gastrointestinal species, has been covered in a number of excellent reviews[1-6] which should be consulted for additional background information. It is proposed here to discuss a limited number of questions concerning the initiation and expression of intestinal immune responses against parasitic organisms and to draw on data from a restricted number of examples. To provide a context for this discussion, a brief outline is given of some of the effector mechanisms known to operate in response to antigenic challenge of the gut. More detailed accounts of these mechanisms are available in this volume (Chapters 1 and 3 [Volume I]) and elsewhere.[5,7,8]

The gastrointestinal tract is exposed to a vast array of potential antigenic moieties, of which a substantial proportion originates from commensal and parasitic organisms. Penetration of the mucosal barrier by these antigens may activate both local and systemic responses. Hosts have evolved a complex system of both immunological and nonimmunological defenses whose function is to limit antigen uptake, maintain the integrity of the epithelial layer, and remove the source of the antigens.

Igs of various isotypes occur within the tissues, associated lymphoid organs, and lumen of the gut. Although the dominant antibody produced is the dimeric secretory form of IgA,[9] this has yet to be identified as a major effector of antiparasite immunity, although its well-documented functions in preventing bacterial adherence, activation of complement, enhancement of mucus trapping, and antibody-dependent cell-mediated cytoxicity (ADCC) of bacteria would seem to fit it for this role.[10-12] In contrast, both IgG isotypes and IgE have been implicated in protective responses against a number of intestinal parasites. Large numbers of IgE-bearing cells and lymphocytes bearing Fc receptors for IgE occur in the gut-associated lymphoid tissue (GALT),[13,14] and these increase during infection with metazoan parasites. IgE is likely to play an important role in mucosal allergic reactions.

T lymphocytes are dispersed throughout the lamina propria and epithelium,[15,16] and precursors of gut T cells are present within Peyer's patches and mesenteric lymph nodes

(MLN). Protective responses to many intestinal parasites are T cell dependent,[17] but the precise roles played by these cells have still to be identified in many cases. The recent development of techniques of isolation and study of gut T cells,[18] which have demonstrated NK (natural killer) and ADCC activity, will allow progress in this field. T lymphoblasts from the GALT are preferentially retained in the intestinal tissues regardless of their antigenic specificity, and this process is enhanced during parasitic infection.[19] GALT T cells are known to play an important role in antibody isotype switching mechanisms, to generate delayed-type skin hypersensitivity (DTH) reactions and to control differentiation and infiltration of a wide variety of other cell populations, e.g., mucosal mast cells (MMC), basophils, eosinophils, and goblet cells.[20-25]

MMC are characteristically associated with gastrointestinal helminth infection, and when triggered by IgE-antigen complexes or by parasite-associated factors, they liberate a wide variety of biologically active materials. Mast cell infiltration is often associated with tissue eosinophilia,[5] and eosinophils release a number of factors (enzymes, leukotrienes, and prostaglandins) which interact directly or indirectly with parasites. There has been renewed interest recently in the effector role of intestinal mucus during parasitic infections and it is now known that goblet cell numbers may increase during infection. Mucus release can be induced by orally presented antigen or immune complexes[26,27] and by several other factors present during infection, so that efficient triggering would be expected under these conditions.

Discussion of effector mechanisms must also include the many pathophysiological changes which occur in the intestine following induction of antiparasite immune responses.[28] These may prove to be the functional end point of complexly induced responses, removing parasites through the physical consequences of fluid secretion, change of intestinal architecture, and increased peristalsis.

IV. EXPERIMENTAL STUDIES IN LABORATORY MODELS

Much of the available information concerning the immune responses evoked by gastrointestinal parasites has been obtained from laboratory models using a variety of rodent hosts. In some cases these models employ parasites that are of direct medical or veterinary significance. In the majority of cases, because of restricted host specificity, it has been necessary to develop models that utilize infections with rodent parasites related or analogous to species of clinical importance.

A. Protozoa

Intestinal protozoa occur commonly in both man and domestic animals. Many species appear to be quite harmless and are regarded as normal intestinal commensals; other species can be severely pathogenic and give rise to acute clinical conditions. Progress in understanding the nature of immune responses to such protozoa has been limited by the availability of manipulable experimental models. Thus, relatively little is known about immunity against *Entamoeba histolytica,* the cause of amebic dysentery, because laboratory studies are largely limited to guinea pigs, hamsters, and neonatal rats and mice. Mouse and rat models have been developed for two other major protozoan diseases, giardiasis and coccidiosis, and these are attracting increasing attention.

1. Giardiasis

Mice are readily infected with *Giardia muris,* a lumen-dwelling, mucosal-adherent protozoan which resembles the human parasite *G. lamblia* in many respects, and develop strong immunity to reinfection once they have controlled an initial infection. The ability to control infection and resist challenge is a thymus-dependent phenomenon, and the increased susceptibility of nude mice can be reversed by adoptive transfer of lymphocytes from normal littermates.[29] Immunity is transferred from immune mothers to their offspring via the milk,[30] where specific anti-*Giardia* IgA and IgG antibodies have been demonstrated.

Although *Giardia* is essentially a lumen-dwelling organism, living attached to epithelial cells, trophozoites do penetrate the epithelium. Electron microscopy (EM) studies have shown that forms invading the Peyer's patches can be phagocytosed by macrophages.[31] Macrophages containing digested *G. muris* were surrounded by lymphoblasts, a situation that clearly suggests a mechanism for efficient antigen uptake and presentation. (This observation has been used to explain the paradox of a luminal parasite initiating immune responses, but it is clear from many sources that uptake of soluble antigens across the epithelium is a normal physiological process and quite capable of eliciting both enteral and systemic responses.) Luminal trophozoites have also been seen in contact with free lymphocytes, although the significance of this observation cannot yet be assessed.

The effectiveness of immunity to an initial *G. muris* infection varies markedly between mouse strains, some (e.g., BALB/c) being relatively resistant and others (e.g., C3H/He) being susceptible and excreting fecal cysts for prolonged periods.[32] In both strains there is good immunity to reinfection once the initial infection has been cleared, and in both, immune mothers transfer protection to their young. No difference in serum levels of parasite-specific IgA or IgG has been detected. In addition, although immunoprecipitation studies with serum antibodies have shown that BALB/c mice selectively recognize certain antigens not "seen" by C3H mice, these antigens were ineffective in vaccination experiments.[33] Thus despite circumstantial evidence for involvement of intestinal antibody in protection (from experiments with suckling young) and from observations on immunodeficient patients, antibody alone cannot effect immunity, and attention has turned to the possible involvement of intestinal inflammatory mechanisms as components of protective immunity. Giardiasis in mice does not cause the serious intestinal pathology associated with infection in man, but nevertheless there is evidence of immune-mediated inflammatory change in the intestine, e.g., villous atrophy and crypt hyperplasia occur at peak infection[34,35] and there is an increase in the numbers of intraepithelial lymphocytes.[34] Infections are chronic in mast cell-deficient W^f/W^f mice but well controlled in normal littermates.[33] However, unlike comparable studies with nematode parasites, resistance has not been restored to W^f/W^f mice by reconstitution with normal bone marrow cells. It may well be that not only does an intestinal defect contribute to chronicity of infection in C3H mice but also that infections may generate a suppressive effect (cf. *Nematospiroides dubius* in mice in Section IV. C). Certainly, removal of chronic primary infections by chemotherapy leaves C3H mice resistant to infection.[36]

2. *Coccidiosis*

Infections with coccidia (intracellular parasites belonging to the genus *Eimeria*) present clinical problems in a number of domestic animals, notably poultry but more recently in pigs, cattle, and sheep. A great deal of experimental data has been gained from studies with fowl, and this will be reviewed in Section V, but this host has certain limitations for immunological investigations; some emphasis has therefore been placed on rodent models. Not only do these allow detailed analytical studies to be undertaken, but they make it possible directly to compare responses to coccidia with those known to operate against other intestinal parasites.

The rat and the mouse can be infected with a variety of species of *Eimeria,* and although each host-parasite system shows characteristic features, a number of common points can be emphasized.[37-41] Primary infections are self-limiting, the duration of infection being determined essentially but not completely by the cycles of asexual division undergone within the cells of the intestinal mucosa. In many strains of hosts, experience of a complete primary infection leaves the host substantially immune to challenge, and this immunity is known to be T cell dependent, being absent in thymus-deficient animals and transferable with thoracic duct or GALT lymphocytes taken from immune animals. Immunity shows a high degree of species specificity in its expression, which suggests that effector mechanisms may involve the direct antiparasite activity of lymphocytes or antibodies rather than the indirect effect of inflammatory components. There is already evidence from other systems (see below) that antibody may play an important role in immunity, and it is significant that strains of mice with low (Biozzi Ab/L) or defective (CBA/N) antibody responsiveness show enhanced primary infections.[42] This interpretation is supported by the fact that although immunity is transferable with serum and with lymphocytes, very large numbers of cells are necessary to effect a significant reduction in oocyst output. The number of lymphocytes required for adoptive transfer of immunity against coccidial infections is at least one order of magnitude higher than that required for transfer of immunity against nematode infections.[37,38,43] Additional though controversial support for a direct antiparasite immunity is provided by observations that immunity can be induced by treatment of mice with a dialyzable transfer factor.[44] To date, however, no clear indication of the nature of the postulated direct antiparasite activity has been proposed, and the involvement of inflammatory changes as effector mechanisms cannot at present be excluded. There is a marked inflammatory response to initial infection with increased numbers of goblet cells, mast cells, and intraepithelial lymphocytes, as well as villous atrophy and crypt hyperplasia; on reinfection, the onset of inflammation is very rapid.[38,45] In addition, it has been shown that mice with defective granulocytes are more susceptible to infection.[42] Whatever effector mechanisms are proposed, they must take into account (1) the intracellular location of the parasite, (2) the nearly complete suppression of reproduction in challenge infections, (3) the similar levels of immunity to challenge in animals with different levels of susceptibility to primary infection, and (4) the evidence from studies in fowl that infective sporozoites can penetrate the epithelium of an immune host and remain viable for a considerable time even though they cannot produce a normal infection in that host.[46]

B. Platyhelminths

Although there are a number of species of Platyhelminthes (flukes and tapeworms) which parasitize the intestines of man and domestic animals, few are of major clinical significance. Many other species, however, use the gastrointestinal tract as a means of entry into the host in order to establish larval or adult infections in other parts of the body. Included within this category are several species of major importance (e.g., *Echinococcus* and *Fasciola*).

There is much evidence from laboratory systems to show that strong immunity is elicited by infection with intestinal platyhelminths, but compared with protozoan and nematode parasites, relatively little is known about the underlying responses. Immunity to adult tapeworms, for example, is known to have a major T cell component,[47,48] and there is evidence that infection provokes infiltration of the mucosa by mast cells and eosinophils.[49] However, the degree of inflammation produced is much less than that associated with nematode infections, and to date, little success has been achieved with the analysis of immunity by adoptive and passive transfers.[50]

More is known of immune mechanisms operating against larval stages which are required to penetrate the intestinal mucosa in order to continue development. Metacercariae of *F. hepatica* are susceptible to an eosinophil-mediated attack in the gut wall, and it is of interest that this phase of immunity functions normally in nude rats.[51] Hexacanth larvae of *Taenia taeniaformis* are also prevented from achieving successful mucosal penetration, and there is good evidence for an effector function of IgA antibody in this response.[52,53] IgG antibodies may also be effective against this initial stage of infection with complement activation playing an important role.

C. Nematoda

Nematodes are relatively large worms characterized by possession of a tough, external, collagenous cuticle. The cuticle is now known to be immunogenic and to carry antigens that may be stage-specific in their expression,[54] there is some limited evidence to show that it may act as a target for protective immune responses.[165] More evidence is available to associate protective immunity with antigens released during metabolism or with antigens released in specific physiological activities such as penetration, feeding, moulting, and reproduction.[55] There is considerable debate as to whether there are specific targets for immune responses against these worms. Immunity is reflected in impaired growth, development, and reproductive activity, which may well reflect immune interference with feeding and/or metabolism, but a major expression of immunity against gut nematodes is their expulsion from the intestine (self- or spontaneous-cure and rapid expulsion).[2] Expulsion is always associated with pathophysiological changes in the intestinal environment, and these may act against worm survival in an essentially nonspecific manner, i.e., be specifically and immunologically induced but be effective against any nematode present at that time.

Infection of mice and rats with the trichuroid nematode *Trichinella spiralis* has been one of the most intensively studied experimental systems and has provided much of our current knowledge concerning immunity operating during acute intestinal infection. The first site of the immune response against *T. spiralis* is the GALT, the small intestine being the initial site of parasitization. The duration of the intestinal phase of a primary infection varies between species and strains of host but is generally between 10 and 20 days.[56] This phase is terminated by an expulsion mechanism induced by antigens associated with the initial larval stages of infection. T lymphocytes play a central role in initiating this mechanism, and hosts that are T cell depleted or thymus deprived exhibit prolonged intestinal infection.[57,58] Infection stimulates the production of a population of rapidly dividing T cells in the lymph node draining the site of infection (MLN), and adoptive transfer experiments have shown that these cells mediate expulsion of worms from the intestine.[59,60] Such cells are preferentially retained in the intestinal mucosa of infected animals. This retention is independent of antigen specificity or of vascular changes in the gut but nevertheless provides an effective localization of mediator cells.[61,62] Prior irradiation of recipients of immune mouse T cells removes their ability to mount an accelerated worm expulsion, but this response is restored when irradiated recipients are given normal bone marrow stem cells.[63] Thus it seems likely that T cells per se are not the direct cause of worm expulsion, and there is strong circumstantial evidence to suggest that the role of T cells is to initiate and focus intestinal inflammatory reactions.[56] In both mice and rats infection is associated with a pronounced infiltration of neutrophils, eosinophils, and mast cells into the intestinal mucosa.[64,65] Further, in the mouse, intestinal mastocytosis can be enhanced by adoptive transfer of MLN cells from immune donors.[66] The infiltration of granulocytes is correlated with an increase in tissue and luminal levels of enzymes associated with these cells, e.g., peroxidases and phospholipases,[67,68] and in the rat, there is a similar correlation between infiltration of mast cells and levels of mast cell products (see below). Architectural and epithelial cell kinetic changes also occur in the mucosa, villous atrophy and crypt hyperplasia being particularly pronounced immediately before worm expulsion occurs.[69] A variety of physiological changes, e. g., enhanced peristalsis, also occur. All of these changes are consistent with the concept that T cell-mediated events initiate and aggravate inflammatory processes. This together with the fact that worms are expelled alive (i.e., are capable of reestablishment if transferred into naive recipients) supports the interpretation of worm expulsion as a nonspecific consequence of gut inflammation.

In the rat it has been proposed that both B and T cells may play a role in worm expulsion, but the role of antibody in immunity to *T. spiralis* is still unresolved.[70] Transfer of immunity with immune serum (assessed by accelerated worm expulsion) has been described,[71] and in one report the isotypes effective in the mouse were identified as IgG1, and IgE.[72] However, these successful transfers were achieved using immunologically competent recipients; transfer of B cell-enriched fractions of immune MLN cells into irradiated recipients resulted only in a reduced fecundity of adult females, implying that active participation by the recipient is necessary for expulsion to occur.[164] To date the only data supporting a direct antiworm effect by Ig came from the work of Jacqueline et al.,[73] who demonstrated that intestinal IgA depressed worm fecundity in vitro.

Much of the present conceptual framework of immunity to intestinal nematodes was laid down by work using the rat *Nippostrongylus brasiliensis* model. This work has been extensively reviewed,[1] and only selected points will be discussed here. An early finding was that immunity to *N. brasiliensis* was associated with pronounced intestinal inflammation[74] and could be transferred to naive recipients with both immune serum and immune lymphocytes.[6] The isotype IgG1 was identified as the effective component in immune serum,[75] other Ig classes being ineffective with T cells being the effective component in immune lymphocytes.[76] Passive transfer into irradiated or suppressed recipients was effective in "damaging" worms but failed to accelerate their expulsion from the intestine. From these and many other observations came the concept that full expression of immunity against *N. brasiliensis* required (1) a T cell-dependent, antiworm antibody (IgG) which could induce cytopathological changes in the worm, (2) a mechanism for allowing antibody to enter the lumen, where the worms lived, and (3) an additional mechanism, inflammatory in nature, which resulted in worm expulsion. A great deal of attention has been focused on the ability of *N. brasiliensis* infections to induce high levels of IgE antibody and to stimulate intense mucosal mastocytosis. These properties, which are shared with other nematodes such as *T. spiralis*, provide the components necessary for immediate hypersensitivity reactions within the mucosa which could account for items 2 and 3 above. A great deal of controversy exists about the relevance of such reactions to immunity in vivo, and many other mechanisms have also been proposed. For example, there is a suggestive correlation between levels of antiworm IgA in the intestine and worm loss.[77,78] Recent evidence, using a radioimmunoassay to measure levels of serum and tissue rat mast cell protease (RMCP II — a component actively released by mast cells) has for the first time shown a direct correlation between MMC activity and worm expulsion, thus reviving the possibility that mast cells play a major role in this process. A similar correlation exists in the expulsion of *T. spiralis* from the rat.[79] In only one system, that of *Trichostrongylus colubriformis* in the guinea pig, is there unequivocal evidence for a role of amines and amine-containing cells (in this case basophils) in the expulsion of nematodes.[22]

A characteristic feature of immunity to both *N. brasiliensis* and *Trichinella spiralis*, particularly in the rat, is the very rapid rejection of secondary infections. In the latter, rapid expulsion (RE) is achieved within a few hours of challenge.[56] In other hosts and for a proportion of challenge worms in rats, expulsion takes place in an accelerated version of the primary response. The kinetics of RE suggest an immediate hypersensitivity (IH) response, but there is little evidence for this at present and some against it, in that drugs which might be expected to block IH do not prevent RE.[80] A role for mucus trapping of worms, preventing establishment, has been proposed for both species.[81] Certainly, goblet cell numbers increase as a result of primary infections, and mucus release is known to be influenced by immunological events. Detailed studies also suggest that immunological factors, at present unspecified, are responsible for rapid changes in ion flux through epithelial cells during RE and for a change in the intestine from net fluid absorption to net secretion.[82,83] Other studies imply that priming for RE requires both a specific immunological component and an intestinal (inflammatory?) component which can be acquired nonspecifically.[84]

Both *N. brasiliensis* and *T. spiralis* are used as models of acute nematode infections, i.e., infections in which the intestinal phase is short lived. *Nematospiroides dubius* in the mouse is, in contrast, used as a model of chronic infections, e.g., those which occur with human hookworms. After infection, *N. dubius* passes through a histotrophic phase within the gut wall before emerging to mature in the lumen. Adult *N. dubius* can survive in mice for 8 months or longer[85] despite evidence under controlled conditions for a potent immunogenicity. A pronounced serum IgG1 hypergammaglobulinemia develops during infection, and although a proportion of the Ig is specific for the adult worm and can passively protect against a challenge larval infection, no effect upon the lumen-dwelling adult stage can be demonstrated.[86,87] A large body of evidence points to the fact that *N. dubius* infections are associated with immunosuppression in the host, reducing responses to a variety of unrelated antigens including other parasites. Recently, it has been shown that antigens of adult *N. dubius* can suppress immune responses to sheep red blood cells (SRBC) both in vitro and in vivo. The in vivo suppression is mediated via cells and may reflect the production by the adult worms of immunomodulatory factors. Immune suppression is a feature of infections with many other intestinal nematodes and may be a mechanism whereby such organisms promote their own survival.

V. EXPERIMENTAL STUDIES IN DOMESTIC ANIMALS

The most important gastrointestinal parasites of domestic animals are the coccidia (protozoans of the genus *Eimeria*) and the gastrointestinal nematodes. Although a variety of other parasites do cause disease in domestic stock, they are less significant economically and much less well studied.

A. Coccidia

Attention will be focused on experimental studies of coccidial infections in fowl. Species of *Eimeria* are pathogenic in many other domestic animals, e.g., pigs, sheep, cattle, and rabbits, but analysis of immune responses is not as well advanced in these hosts. Several species can infect the fowl; of these, the most intensively studied have been those associated with the greatest patholoy (e.g., *E. tenella, E. necatrix, E. maxima, and E. acervulina*). Although the immune response to these species shows strict specificity and there are real differences between them in the details of immunity stimulated by infection, it is possible to discuss this immunity in general terms. As in the rodent systems discussed above, primary infections are self-limiting and immunity is expressed most strongly in terms of challenge infections. Thymectomy and bursectomy have been used in attempts to identify the effectors of immunity but with equivocal results.[88] Successful transfer of immunity has been achieved using spleen cells and peripheral blood lymphocytes[89] but not with cecal tonsil cells, and there was a correlation, using concurrent priming with human RBC as a marker antigen, between the ability of cells to transfer both antibody and cell-mediated responses to human RBC and the ability to affect oocyst output. Together with the data from thymectomy/bursectomy experiments, these results imply that both antiparasite antibody (T dependent) and a T cell-mediated cellular response are necessary for full expression of immunity. Several factors point to an involvement of IgA antibody in immunity. Infection with *E. tenella* causes an increase in the number of IgA cells at the site of infection, and a selective increase in IgA within the cecal lumen. Intestinal contents, taken from the ceca of infected chickens had antiparasite activity in vitro.[90] Davis and Porter[91] proposed that in vivo IgA antisporozoite antibody present in mucus would impede the penetration of epithelial cells and thus expose the parasite to damage from nonspecific (enzymatic?) components of the cecal lumen. Many sporozoites would break free from the antibodies and penetrate cells but would fail to develop further. The paradox that sporozoites are known to invade epithelia of immune hosts and remain sufficiently viable to reinfect naive hosts on transfer was explained by proposing that damaged sporozoites were able to recover if removed from the immune environment. This suggestion is consistent to some extent with other observations which show that B-deficient chickens express good immunity to challenge;[88] i.e., there must be another, possibly cell-mediated, response operative within the mucosa itself.

The nature of this latter response is undefined. It is known that parasites can be phagocytosed by macrophages and heterophils[92,93] in vitro but infectivity is not necessarily lost. Furthermore, sporozoites can enter intraepithelial lymphocytes for the initial stages of infection.[94] Whether the fate of the intracellular phase can be altered by immunity at this stage has still to be resolved. Infection does result in infiltration of the mucosa by a variety of inflammatory cells, but unlike the situation in rodent hosts, infection does not stimulate a pronounced mastocytosis.[95] Challenge infections given to immune chickens elicit an extremely rapid (within 7 hr) infiltration of heterophils and lymphocytes into the mucosa, and this is paralleled by an equally rapid rise in number of circulating leukocytes.[96] Thus there is an intestinal response which could be correlated with the highly specific and highly efficient resistance known to exist against reinfection, but whether this correlation is more than contingent remains to be seen.

B. Nematoda

Although laboratory studies have provded many useful insights into the initiation and expression of immune responses against intestinal nematodes, it is not always easy to relate them directly to the results of comparable work with domestic animals; nevertheless there are a number of significant similarities. Early concepts of intestinal effector mechanisms against intestinal nematodes were heavily influenced by the work of Stoll[97] and Stewart[98] on self-cure in sheep, which focused attention on immediate hypersensitivity responses as the cause of inflammatory changes inimical to worm survival in the intestine. Much subsequent work has been concerned with the investigation of the detailed immunological responses underlying self-cure and other forms of resistance.

The roles of lymphocytes in mediating the response to gut-dwelling nematodes of domestic animals are still largely unresolved, although recently, following the adoptive transfer techniques used so successfully in laboratory models, Smith et al.[99] have shown that the transfer of large numbers of lymphoblasts collected from the gastric lymph of sheep infected with *Haemonchus contortus,* was successful in generating resistance to reinfection in histocompatible hosts. The establishment of the sheep intestinal nematode *Trichostrongylus colubriformis* in laboratory guinea pigs has shown that the adoptive transfer of immunity with MLN cells is possible, although successful transfer was dependent upon the age of cell donors, the level of infection of the recipients, and the number of cells transferred.[100]

Sheep infected with *H. contortus* or *T. colubriformis* exhibit increased levels of parasite-specific antibodies at their respective infection sites, the majority being of the IgA isotype.[101,102] Increased levels of parasite-specific IgA have been demonstrated in sheep immune to *T. colubriformis,*[103] and an increase in IgA specific for *Ostertagia circumcincta* was noted in the lymph of sheep challenged with large numbers of larvae.[104]

Morever, substantial increases in IgA antibody and IgA blast cells in lymph draining the gastric mucosa of sheep repeatedly infected with *O. circumcincta* have been reported.[105] Indeed, these studies and others suggest that IgA production in the intestine of sheep may have a strong protective role.

A number of reports have been made concerning hyperplasia of mucus-secreting cells of domestic animals infected with certain gut nematodies, and although there is no direct evidence of their involvement in immune responses, in the cases of *T. vitrinus*,[106] *Oesophagostomum columbianum*,[107,108] and *H. contortus*[109] infections of sheep, there is evidence to suggest a correlation with resistance. Bearing in mind the technical difficulties encountered when analyzing parasite-specific antibodies in mucus, Dobson[107,110] has reported high levels of parasite-specific antibodies in mucus from intestinal extracts from *O. columbianum*-infected sheep. Mast cell involvement in antiparasite responses of domestic animals has received little investigation, although globule leukocytes which are thought to be related to mast cells[111] have often been observed in resistant animals.[112] Eosinophil infiltration of the mucosa is a characteristic of many gastrointestinal nematode parasites of ruminants, although not necessarily associated with resistance.[107,113-116]

VI. IMMUNE RESPONSES IN MAN

Although there have been many descriptions of systemic responses to infection with intestinal parasites in man, it is difficult to assess the significance of these responses either in relation to the course of infection as seen in man or in relation to the data gained from studies in experimental animals. For example, serological responses, being easily examined, have been well documented, and it is clear the intestinal infections elicit systemic antibodies capable of reacting with antigens prepared from the parasite concerned.[117] Such antibodies may be useful diagnostically, but their relationship to immunity is often obscure. Similarly, intestinal infections prime for DTH responses, but, again, the relationship to immunity is unclear. Attention will therefore be focused here on responses that are relevant to immunity or which can be interpreted in the light of experimental data.

A. Giardiasis

Infection produces a wide clinical spectrum, ranging from an asymptomatic carrier condition to severe malabsorption, diarrhea, and weight loss. Acute symptomatic episodes have been interpreted as the by-products of protective intestinal responses; chronic infections and disease have been explained by a failure to mount such responses effectively. Giardiasis is common in immunodeficient, hypogammaglobulinemic individuals[118] who frequently show villous atrophy, crypt hyperplasia, and impaired epithelial absorption. Reduced or absent circulating IgA is a feature of this group, and it may be assumed that intestinal IgA is equally affected. Giardiasis does, however, also occur in immunologically normal individuals, who may then show similar intestinal changes, suggesting that the pathology is the result of cell-mediated, mucosal responses, an interpretation consistent with experimental data (see Section IV.A.1). Biopsies have shown eosinophilic infiltration into the duodenal lamina propria.[119] Experimental data[120,121] suggested that an effective immunity could develop in man after a single exposure to infection, but not all subjects tested developed immunity.

B. Intestinal Nematodes

Nematodes are the most prevalent intestinal parasites; for example, the large roundworm, *Ascaris lumbricoides*, occurs in an estimated 1250 million people, and other species (such as hookworms and *Trichuris*) are almost as abundant.[122] Little is known of protective immunity against these parasites; indeed, there is circumstantial evidence (the ease of reinfection after chemotherapy) which suggests that immunity is very inefficient. However, rates of infection do tend to stabilize or decline with increasing age. Infections are also associated with marked immunological phenomena, of which elevated levels of serum IgE, allergic symptoms, and blood eosinophilia are the best known.[123] The mechanisms by which worms elicit these responses in man are unknown, but it can be assumed that they are similar to those which operate in experimental animals (see below) and are related to the presence of powerful allergens in components of the worms' bodies.[124] The involvement of a tissue migratory phase during development may also be an important factor, as infections with *Trichuris,* which develops directly in the large intestine, are not associated with these phenomena. Little is known of intestinal responses to infection; jejunal biopsies from patients infected with hookworms have shown edema and cellular infiltration but not villous atrophy. It is interesting that because of difficulties with fixation, nothing is yet known of MMC responses in human nematode infections despite these cells being a characteristic feature of such infections in other hosts.[125]

One of the most intriguing immunological puzzles concerning intestinal nematode infections in man centers around the phenomenon of hyperinfection with *Strongyloides stercoaalis.* This skin-penetrating species lives as a parthenogenetic female in the small intestine. Infections are associated with raised IgE and eosinophilia, but in a majority of cases cause few overt symptoms. However, infections appear to be remarkably persistent even at very low levels and can flare up when the host is suppressed immunologically. Under these circumstances the host becomes massively and sometimes fatally infected by larval parasites which become disseminated through the whole body.[126] The origin of these larvae may be residual adults within the intestine; if this is so, then immunosuppression must both remove inhibitory influences upon worm reproduction and facilitate tissue invasion by larvae. Nothing is yet known of these phenomena in man, although related problems have been studied using animal models.[127]

VII. IMMUNOLOGICAL CONSEQUENCES OF INTESTINAL INFECTION

Not all of the immune responses associated with parasitic infections in the intestine can be positively related to protective immunity, and some indeed are positively harmful to the host in certain circumstances. In circumventing the defense mechanisms of the host, parasites clearly run the risk of initiating immunopathological responses which may act to their detriment by reducing the overall fitness of the host. Phenomenological descriptions of parasite infections have frequently been concerned with responses of this type, and a number of them have proved to be of considerable interest to workers in other immunological fields, providing models by which particular responses can be readily induced and studied. Four such responses are briefly discussed below.

A. IgE

One of the outstanding features of gastrointestinal helminth infections is their capacity to stimulate the production of high levels of circulating IgE antibody in the host. Indeed, much of the information now available concerning the regulation of production and function of this isotype has been derived from studies using IgE responses generated by parasitic infection. IgE antibody is characterized by prolonged tissue fixation via high-affinity binding of its Fc region to receptors in the plasma membranes of cells such as mast cells and basophils and by its major role in immediate hypersensitivity reactions. The accumulation of amine-containing cells in the intestinal mucosa during helminth infection may indicate a protective role for IgE through its participation in inflammatory events.[128] Parasite-specific IgE may also participate in ADCC reactions,[129] although little is known concerning the way in which IgE is transported into the intestine (see Section VI.B) or the nature of IgE-cell interactions along the gastrointestinal tract. The ability of helminths to evoke IgE production so successfully was initially considered to be a property of the intact, living organism, but it is now known that many species contain potent allergens which can be used in isolation. The allergens of *Ascaris* spp. have been studied particularly used in a wide variety of experimental systems.[130]

In addition to parasite-specific IgE, helminth infections have been shown to potentiate the production of IgE against unrelated, nonparasite antigens. Elevated total IgE levels have been described during infection with several species of both nematodes and platyhelminths,[128] but detailed analysis of the phenomenon is restricted to the rat *Nippostrongylus* model. T cell involvement is essential for the production of both parasite-specific and nonspecific IgE,[131-133] and both an "IgE-potentiating factor" and an "IgE-suppressive factor" have been shown to be released from MLN cells taken from rats infected with this nematode.[133,134] B cells taken from the MLN of infected rats release a factor termed "IgE B cell-generating factor" when activated by cross-linking of receptors either by antigen or by anti-IgE.[135,136] This factor was found to increase the proportion of cells expressing both surface IgE and IgM, suggesting that it induced IgM-bearing cells to express surface IgE.[136]

The role of nonspecific IgE production during helminth infection is still open to debate. Competitive inhibition of amine-containing cell surface receptors by nonspecific IgE may be a mechanism whereby specific allergic responses are reduced.[128] In this context it is interesting to speculate on the importance of tolerance, suppressor T cells, idiotype, and isotype suppression in the regulation of parasite-specific IgE synthesis and their relationship to parasite survival in the gastrointestinal tract.

B. MMC

Gastrointestinal parasites, most particularly nematodes, induce a pronounced infiltration of the gut mucosa by a distinctive population of amine-containing cells, the MMC. The presence of such cells, which occur in other disease conditions as well, is clearly of significance when potential pathological sequelae are being considered, and in consequence these cells have been intensively studied. Much of what is now known about this important subset of mast cells has stemmed from parasitological observations. Infections have provided both a source of cells and a means of analyzing the conditions necessary for their production and differentiation. For example, infections with *Trichinella spiralis* in nude and normal mice have confirmed that MMC are heavily thymus dependent and distinct in this respect from connective tissue mast cells.[137] Preparative techniques, using mucosal tissue taken from rats infected with *N. brasiliensis,* have allowed the isolation and purification of MMC and thus the analysis of their mediators and their pharmacological properties.[138,139] Although MMC are similar in many respects to connective tissue cells, there are important differences in the composition of their granules, which in rat MMC contain less strongly sulfated glycosaminoglycans and less monoamine and have distinctive proteases. In addition, their responses to ionophores and antiallergic compounds also differ from other mast cells,[5,125] and release of mediators can be by continuous secretion rather than by exocytosis. Identification of a characteristic protease in rat MMC (rat mast cell protease II) and development of a radioimmunoassay for its measurement have made it possible for the first time to correlate MMC function with immune responses to intestinal parasites[79] rather than attempt to draw conclusions from static histological data. In the past, such data have generated considerable confusion concerning the functional relation of MMC to worm expulsion, confusion that has not really been dispelled by the use of mutant mice such as W/W^v which lack normal MMC responses. Measurement of rat mast cell protease II shows that mediator release coincides with worm expulsion and strengthens the hypothesis that mucosal inflammatory changes do contribute to protective immunity against intestinal helminths. This contribution is, however, probably not essential, as immunity can be expressed in the absence of functional MMC.[6]

The origin of MMC has long been disputed, but data from parasitological studies have consistently pointed to a T cell-dependent differentiation from bone marrow precursors. Several workers using rats and mice infected with *N. brasiliensis* or *T. spiralis* showed that mucosal mastocytosis could be accelerated by passive transfer of immune serum or adoptive transfer of immune lymphocytes (T cells),[6] although in all cases, infection with the living parasite was necessary to initiate the response. Genetic studies in mice[140] showed that the MMC response to *T. spiralis* was strain dependent; analysis, including the use of radiation chimeras, indicating that the level of responsiveness achieved was controlled by genetic mechanisms expressed through a population of bone marrow cells which required T cell help for their differentiation into MMC. Both bone marrow origin and T cell dependency of MMC have recently been confirmed experimentally,[141,142] the latter work showing that MMC precursors differentiate and proliferate in response to the release of interleukin 3 from a population of antigen-stimulated, gut mucosal T cells.

Despite the considerable progress that has been made in this field, many interesting problems remain. For example, MMC possess receptors for IgE and release mediators when they are cross-linked by IgE-antigen complexes in the normal way. However, evidence gained initially from studies in *N. brasiliensis*-infected rats showed that MMC transport IgE into the mucosa both on their surface and cytoplasmically.[143] The significance of this observation has yet to be fully understood. The clinical significance of MMC in a variety of pathological conditions involving inflammatory changes in the human intestine is only now being evaluated, as earlier studies failed to use histological techniques adequate for MMC identification.

C. Eosinophils

The eosinophil, long considered to be an enigmatic cell, is now known to play an important role in inflammatory reactions of immunological origin, modulating the activities of a variety of other cell types and contributing to both protective and pathological responses.[23] Parasitologically oriented studies have contributed significantly to the analysis of eosinophil function. Peripheral blood eosinophilia is characteristic of many helminth infections, and laboratory infections in rodent hosts provide a convenient source of cells as well as models for investigating aspects of the control and regulation of eosinophil kinetics. Although eosinophilia is particularly pronounced in infections in which worms are located parenterally, it is also characteristic of gastrointestinal infections, e.g., *Ascaris* and hookworms in man and comparable species in rodents. These nematodes have preliminary parenteral migratory phases, but it is known from experimental studies with other species such as *T. spiralis* and the wholly intestinal species *Nematospiroides dubius* and *Trichostrongylus colubriformis* that enteral stages alone can generate a marked eosinophilia.[144-146]

Intestinal infections are also associated with eosinophil infiltration of the mucosa, a phenomenon that is thymus dependent.[147] The proven functional interrelationships of mast cells and eosinophils suggest that mucosal infiltration of the two cell types may be causally connected, but technical difficulties have so far precluded any direct studies with MMC and eosinophils. As with mastocytosis, the correlation of mucosal eosinophilia with protective responses against the eliciting infection has been the subject of much speculation. Although it is now well established that eosinophils can participate in IgG- and IgE-mediated ADCC reactions against helminths in vitro,[23] there is as yet no direct evidence that these occur during intestinal infections. It is, however, possible that direct interactions of this type may affect responses against the intramucosal stages of worms such as *N. dubius* and *Hymenolepis nana.* Eosinophil infiltration of the mucosa may be involved in the mediation of immunity against intestinal worms via the release of enzymes and inflammatory mediators, and the effects of these directly upon the worms themselves or indirectly via effects upon the intestinal environment. Circumstantial support for this suggestion comes from the measurement of myeloperoxidases and phospholipase enzymes during infection[28,68] and the fact that treatment of infected hosts with antieosinophil serum decreases resistance to worms which are entirely luminal in location.[148]

An important corollary of eosinophil invasion of organs is the possibility that tissues may be damaged as eosinophils degranulate and release their mediator substances.[149] Nothing is known at present of the potential for pathological change in the intestines of patients carrying chronic helminth infections, although the frequency of eosinophilic infiltration may well be very high.

Compared with purely immunological responses, little is known at present concerning the genetic control of inflammatory responses involving cells such as the eosinophil. Recent studies involving both conventional antigens and intestinal parasitic infections have shown that genetic variation does exist in the ability of mice to mount eosinophil responses[150,151] and have provided models in which the mode of expression of genetic control can be analyzed.

D. Tolerance and Immunosuppression

The induction of systemic tolerance to antigens presented along the gastrointestinal tract is a well-documented phenomenon,[152,153] although ongoing local responses, e.g., IgA production, may continue locally. It has been postulated that after presentation of antigens via the gut, antigen-specific suppressor T cells may appear sequentially in the Peyer's patches, MLN, thoracic duct lymph, and spleen, a sequence which suggests the development of such cells at mucosal sites and migration to systemic lymphoid tissue.[153,154]

Immunodepression is a prominent feature of many acute parasitic infections of the gut, including *Trichinella spiralis, Nippostrongylus brasiliensis,* and *E. nieschulzi.*[155-158] In the case of the chronic infection of *Nematospiroides dubius* in mice,[159] the adult worm which lives in the lumen is known to suppress the normal response mounted against a number of heterologous antigens. Indeed, it is now known that the suppression observed against SRBC response is mediated by a suppressor cell population which can be generated by direct administration of an adult antigen preparation.[160] Recently, it has been demonstrated that the immunity generated by the larval stages of the parasite can be suppressed by the transfer of adult worms into the host by laparotomy.[161] Thus in this situation the immunodepression observed is of direct benefit to the parasite, since it interferes with protective immunity.

The immunodepression associated with *N. dubius* is active against other gastrointestinal parasites, and analysis of this phenomenon has revealed a number of important phenomena.[162] In concurrent infections of mice with *N. dubius* and *T. spiralis* the normal immune response of the latter is considerably delayed. In addition, the presence of *N. dubius* prevents the enhanced localization of mesenteric node lymphoblasts that is so characteristic of *T. spiralis* infection;[61] i.e., *N. dubius* influences local intestinal responses to infection. Mice harboring *N. dubius* appear to be incapable of expressing anti-*T. spiralis* immunity when adoptive transfer of *T. spiralis*-immune lymphocytes is given, but this inhibition is removed rapidly when the *N. dubius* is cleared from the intestine by chemotherapy, a phenomenon that is difficult to relate to the activity of nonspecific suppressor activity unless this is of very short duration.

The degree of suppression exerted by *N. dubius* is a characteristic of particular parasite-mouse strain combinations; i.e., it is influenced by host genetic factors. Major histocompatibility complex-controlled dose-dependent immune suppression of specific responses has recently been demonstrated in *Trichinella* infections in mice.[163] In animals infected with large numbers of worms, expulsion of worms from the intestine was delayed, and lymphocyte responsiveness to parasite antigen depressed; these effects were modulated by H-2 linked genes.

These examples serve to illustrate that gut parasites are capable of generating both local and generalized immunosuppression, which in some cases has been shown to benefit the parasite. However, the relationship between this suppression and the generation of classical oral tolerance remains to be discovered.

VIII. CONCLUSIONS

The aim of this chapter has been to show that analysis of the immunological responses initiated by infections with gastrointestinal parasites has not only applied significance in terms of prophylaxis but also fundamental interest in shedding light upon the capacity of the gastrointestinal tract to respond adaptively to antigenic stimulation. The variety of parasitic organisms capable of life within the gut and the variety of their associations with the host provide a series of manipulable model systems with which both applied and fundamental questions can be studied. Certain systems provide almost unique opportunities for analysis of immunological function and inflammatory response, and the potential of these systems has yet to be fully realized. Their value lies not only in their manipulability but also in their representation of "real" situations in which the scientist has the opportunity to study the integrated responses of intact hosts to natural forms of gastrointestinal antigen stimulation. The goals of such work are the greater understanding of adaptive immunity in the intestine and the possibility of changing the balance of host-parasite relationships in man and his domestic stock, a balance which at present is often overwhelmingly in favor of the parasite.

ACKNOWLEDGMENTS

The authors wish to acknowledge with gratitude the financial support that both have received from the British Medical Research Council.

REFERENCES

1. Ogilvie, B. M. and Love, R. J., Co-operation between antibodies and cells in immunity to a nematode parasite, *Transplant. Rev.*, 19, 147, 1974.
2. Wakelin, D., Immunity to intestinal parasites, *Nature (London)*, 273, 617, 1978.
3. Catty, D. and Ross, I. N., Immunological aspects of infection with gastrointestinal parasites (protozoa and nematodes), in *Immunology of the Gastrointestinal Tract*, Asquith, P., Ed., Churchill Livingstone, Edinburgh, 1979, 246.
4. Mitchell, G. F., Responses to infection with metazoan and protozoan parasites in mice, *Adv. Immunol.*, 28, 451, 1979.
5. Befus, D. and Bienenstock, J., Factors involved in symbiosis and host resistance at the mucosa-parasite interface, *Prog. Allergy*, 31, 76, 1982.
6. Miller, H. R. P., The protective mucosal response against gastrointestinal nematodes in ruminants and laboratory animals, *Vet. Immunol. Immunopathol.*, 6, 167, 1984.

7. Porter, R. and Knight, J., *Immunology of the Gut,* CIBA Foundation Symposium 46, Exerpta Medica, Amsterdam, 1977.
8. Strober, W., Hanson, L. A., and Sell, K. W., Eds., *Recent Advances in Mucosal Immunity,* Raven Press, New York, 1982.
9. Shearman, D. J. C., Parkin, D. M., and McClelland, D. B. C., The demonstration and function of antibodies in the gastrointestinal tract, *Gut,* 13, 483, 1972.
10. Tomasi, T. B., Jr. and Bienenstock, J., Secretory immunoglobulins, in *Advances in Immunology,* Vol. 9, Dixon, F. J. and Kunkel, H. G., Eds., Academic Press, New York, 1968.
11. Lowell, G. H., Smith, L. F., Griffiss, J. M., and Brandt, B. L., IgA-dependant monocyte mediated, antibacterial activity, *J. Exp. Med.,* 152, 452, 1980.
12. Tagliabaue, A., Nencioni, L., Villa, L., Keren, D. F., Lowell, G. H., and Boraschi, D., Antibody-dependant cell mediated antibacterial activity of intestinal lymphocytes with secretory IgA, *Nature (London),* 306, 184, 1983.
13. Durkin, H. G. and Waksman, B. H., High concentrations of IgE and IgA bearing cells in Peyer's patches of germ free rats, *Fed. Proc., Fed. Am. Soc. Exp. Biol.,* 38, 1081, 1979.
14. Yodoi, J. and Ishizaka, K., Lymphocytes bearing Fc receptors for IgE. IV. Formation of IgE binding factor by rat T lymphocytes, *J. Immunol.,* 124, 1322, 1980.
15. Arnaud-Battandier, F., Immunologic characteristics of isolated gut mucosal lymphoid cells, in *Recent Advances in Mucosal Immunity,* Strober, W., Hanson, L. A., and Sell, K. W., Eds., Raven Press, New York, 1982, 289.
16. Parrott, D. M. V., The characterization of lymphocyte populations in the small intestine, in, *Mechanisms of Gastrointestinal Inflammation,* Chadwick, V. S., Ed., Smith, Kline & French, Oxford, 1984, 1.
17. Mitchell, G. F., T cell-dependant effects in parasitic infection and disease, in *Immunology 80: Progress in Immunology,* Vol. 4, Fougereau, M. and Dausset, J., Eds., Academic Press, London, 1980, 794.
18. Davies, M. D. J. and Parrott, D. M. V., Preparation and purification of lymphocytes from the
19. Parrott, D. M. V. and Wilkinson, P. C., Lymphocyte locomotion and migration, *Prog. Allergy,* 28, 193, 1981.
20. Ferguson, A. and McDonald, T. T., Effects of local delayed hypersensitivity on the small intestine, in *Immunology of the Gut,* Ferguson, A. and MacSween, R. M., Eds., Elsevier/North-Holland, Amsterdam, 1977, 305.
21. Elson, C. O., Heck, J. A., and Strober, W., T cell regulation of murine IgA synthesis, *J. Exp. Med.,* 149, 632, 1979.
22. Askenase, P. W., Immunopathology of parasitic diseases: involvement of basophils and mast cells, *Springer Semin. Immunopathol.,* 2, 417, 1980.
23. Mahmoud, A. A. F. and Austen, K. F., Eds., *The Esinophil in Health and Disease,* Grune & Stratton, New York, 1980.
24. Strober, W. and Kauranishi, H., Regulation of IgA production, in *Mechanisms of Gastrointestinal Inflammation,* Chadwick, V. S., Ed., Smith, Kline & French, Oxford, 1984, 9.
25. Jarrett, E. E. E. and Haig, D. M., Mucosal mast cells *in vivo* and *in vitro, Immunol. Today,* 5, 115, 1984.
26. Forster, J. F., Intestinal mucins in health and disease, *Digestion,* 17, 234, 1978.
27. Lake, A. M., Bloch, K. J., Neutra, M. R., and Walker, W. A., Intestinal goblet cell mucous release. II. *In vivo* stimulation by antigen in the immunized rat, *J. Immunol.,* 122, 234, 1978.
28. Castro, G. A., Spatial and temporal integration of host responses to intestinal stages of *Trichinella spiralis:* retro and prospective views, in *Biochemistry of Parasites and Host-Parasite Relationships,* Van den Bossche, H., Ed., Elsvier/North Holland, Amsterdam, 1976, 307.
29. Stevens, D. P., Giardiasis: immunity, immunopathology and immunodiagnosis, in *Immunology of Parasitic Infections,* 2nd ed., Cohen, S. and Warren, K. S., Eds., Blackwell Scientific, London, 1982, chap. 9.
30. Stevens, D. P. and Frank, D. M., Local immunity in mouse giardiasis: is milk protective at the expense of maternal gut?, *Trans. Assoc. Am. Phys.,* 91, 268, 1978.
31. Owen, R. L., Allen, C. L., and Stevens, D. P., Phagocytosis of *Giardia muris* by macrophages in Peyer's patch epithelium in mice, *Infect. Immun.,* 33, 591, 1981.
32. Roberts-Thomson, I. C. and Mitchell, G. F., Giardiasis in mice. I. Prolonged infections in certain mouse strains and hypothymic (nude) mice, *Gastroenterology,* 75, 42, 1978.
33. Erlich, J. H., Anders, R. F., Roberts-Thomson, I. C., Schrader, J. W., and Mitchell, G. F., An examination of differences in serum antibody specificities and hypersensitivity reactions as contributing factors to chronic infection with the intestinal protozoan parasite, *Giardia muris,* in mice, *Aust. J. Exp. Biol. Med. Sci.,* 61(Part 5), 599, 1983.

34. MacDonald, T. T. and Ferguson, A., Small intestinal epithelial cell kinetics and protozoal infection in mice, *Gastroenterology,* 74, 496, 1978.
35. Brett, S. J. and Cox, F. E. G., Immunological aspects of *Giardia muris* and *Spironucleus muris* infections in inbred and outbred strains of laboratory mice: a comparative study, *Parasitology,* 85, 85, 1982.
36. Underdown, B. J., Roberts-Thomson, I. C., Anders, R. F., and Mitchell, G. F., Giardiasis in mice: studies on the characteristics of chronic infection in CH3/He mice, *J. Immunol.,* 126, 669, 1981.
37. Liburd, E. M., Armstrong, W. D., and Mahart, J. L., Immunity to the protozoan parasite *Eimeria nieschulzi* in inbred CD-F rats, *Cell Immunol.,* 7, 444, 1973.
38. Ogilvie, B. M. and Rose, M. E., The response of the host to some parasites of the small intestine: coccidia and nematodes, *Inserm,* 72, 237, 1977.
39. Klesius, P. H. and Hinds, S. E., Strain-dependant differences in murine susceptibility to coccidia, *Infect. Immun.,* 26, 1111, 1979.
40. Mesfin, G. M. and Bellamy, J. E. C., The thymic dependence of immunity to *Eimeria falciformis* var. *pragensis* in mice, *Infect. Immun.,* 23, 460, 1979.
41. Rose, M. E., Hesketh, P., Ogilvie, B. M., and Festing, M. F. W., Failure of nude (athymic) rats to become resistant to re-infection with the intestinal coccidian parasite *Eimeria nieschulzi* or the nematode *Nippostrongylus brasilensis, Parasite Immunol.,* 1, 125, 1979.
42. Rose, M. E., Owen, D. G., and Hesketh, P., Susceptibility to coccidiosis: effect of strain of mouse on reproduction of *Eimeria vermiformis, Parasitology,* 88, 45, 1984.
43. Rose, M. E., Hesketh, P., and Wakelin, D., Unpublished data, 1980.
44. Klesius, P. H., Elston, A. L., Chambers, W. H., and Fundberg, H. H., Resistance to coccidiosis (*Eimeria ferrisi*) in C57BL/6 mice: effects of immunization and transfer factor, *Clin. Immunol. Immunopathol.,* 12, 143, 1979.
45. Rose, M. E. and Hesketh, P., Coccidiosis: T-lymphocyte dependent effects of infection with *Eimeria nieschulzi* in rats, *Vet. Immunol. Immunopathol.,* 3, 499, 1982.
46. Rose, M. E. and Hesketh, P., Immunity to coccidiosis stages of the life cycle of *Eimeria maxima* which induce and are affected by the response of the host, *Parasitology,* 73, 25, 1976.
47. Isaak, D. A., Jacobson, R. H., and Reed, N. D., Thymus dependence of tapeworm (*Hymenolepis diminuta*) elimination from mice, *Infect. Immun.,* 12, 1478, 1975.
48. Hindsbo, O., Andreassen, J., and Ruitenberg, J., Immunological and histopathological reactions of the rat against the tapeworm, *Hymenolepis diminuta* and the effects of anti-thymocyte serum, *Parasite Immunol.,* 4, 59, 1982.
49. Andreassen, J., Hindsbo, O., and Ruitenberg, E. J., *Hymenolepis diminuta* infections in congenitally athymic (nude) mice: worm kinetics and intestinal histopathology, *Immunology,* 34, 105, 1978.
50. Hopkins, C. A., Immunity and *Hymenolepis diminuta,* in *Biology of the Tapeworm Hymenolepis diminuta,* Arai, H., Ed., Academic Press, New York, 1980, 551.
51. Doy, T. G. and Hughes, D. L., Evidence for two distinct mechanisms of resistance in the rat to reinfection with *Fasciola hepatica, Int. J. Parasitol.,* 12, 357, 1982.
52. Musoke, A. J., Williams, J. F., Leid, R. W., and Williams, C. S. F., The immunological response of the rat to infection with *Taenia taeniaeformis.* IV. Immunoglobulins involved in passive transfer of resistance from mother to offspring, *Immunology,* 29, 845, 1975.
53. Lloyd, S. and Soulsby, E. J. L., The role of IgA immunoglobulins in the passive transfer of protection to *Taenia taeniaeformis* in the mouse, *Immunology,* 34, 939, 1978.
54. Maizels, R. M., Phillipp, M., and Ogilvie, B. M., Molecules on the surface of parasitic nematodes as probes of the immune response to infection, *Immunol. Rev.,* 61, 109, 1982.
55. Mitchell, G. F. and Anders, R. F., Parasite antigens and their immunogenicity in infected hosts, in *The Antigens,* Vol. 6, Sela, M., Ed., Academic Press, New York, 1982, 69.
56. Wakelin, D. and Denham, D. A., The immune response, in *Trichinella and Trichinosis,* Campbell, W. C., Ed., Plenum Press, New York, 1983, 265.
57. Walls, R. S., Carter, R. L., Leuchers, E., and Davies, A. J. S., The immunopathology of trichinosis in T cell deficient mice, *Clin. Exp. Immunol.,* 13, 231, 1973.
58. Ruitenberg, E. J. and Steerenberg, P. A., Intestinal phase of *Trichinella spiralis* in congenitally athymic (nude) mice, *J. Parasitol.,* 60, 1056, 1974.
59. Grencis, R. K. and Wakelin, D., Short lived, dividing cells mediate adoptive transfer of immunity to *Trichinella spiralis* in mice. I. Availability of cells in primary and secondary infections in relation to cellular changes in the mesenteric lymph node, *Immunology,* 46, 443, 1982.
60. Wakelin, D., Grencis, R. K., and Donachie, A. M., Short lived, dividing cells mediate adoptive transfer of immunity to *Trichinella spiralis* in mice. II. *In vivo* characteristics of the cells, *Immunology,* 46, 451, 1982.

61. Rose, M. L., Parrott, D. M. V., and Bruce, R. G., Migration of lymphoblasts to the small intestine. II. Divergent migration of mesenteric and peripheral immunoblasts to sites of inflammation in the mouse, *Cell. Immunol.*, 27, 36, 1976.
62. Ottaway, C. A., Manson-Smith, D. F., Bruce, R. G., and Parrott, D. M. V., Regional blood flow and the localization of lymphoblasts in the small intestine of the mouse. II. The effect of a primary enteric infection with *Trichinella spiralis, Immunology,* 41, 963, 1980.
63. Wakelin, D. and Wilson, M. M., Immunity to *Trichinella spiralis* in irradiated mice, *Int. J. Parasitol.*, 10, 37, 1980.
64. Grove, D. I., Hamburger, J., and Warren, K. S., Kinetics of immunological responses, resistance to reinfection and pathological reactions to infection with *Trichinella spiralis, J. Infect. Dis.*, 136, 562, 1977.
65. Ruitenberg, E. J. and Elgersma, A., Response of intestinal globule leucocytes in the mouse during a *Trichinella spiralis* infection and its independence of intestinal mast cells, *Br. J. Exp. Pathol.*, 60, 246, 1979.
66. Alizadeh, H. and Wakelin, D., Mechanism of rapid expulsion of *Trichinella spiralis* from mice, in *Trichinellosis,* Kim, C. W., Ruitenberg, E. J., and Teppema, J. S., Eds., Reedbooks, Chertsey, 1981, 81.
67. Castro, G. A., Roy, S. A., and Stockstill, R. D., *Trichinella spiralis:* peroxidase activity in isolated cells from rat intestine, *Exp. Parasitol.*, 36, 307, 1974.
68. Larsh, J. E., Ottolenghi, A., and Weatherly, N. F., *Trichinella spiralis:* Phospholipase in challenged mice and rats, *Exp. Parasitol.*, 36, 299, 1975.
69. Manson-Smith, D. F., Bruce, R. G., and Parrott, D. M. V., Villous atrophy and expulsion of intestinal *Trichinella spiralis* are mediated by T-cells, *Cell Immunol.*, 47, 285, 1979.
70. Crum, E. D., Despommier, D. D., and McGregor, D. D., Immunity to *Trichinella spiralis.* I. Transfer of resistance by two classes of lymphocytes, *Immunology,* 33, 787, 1977.
71. Love, R. J., Ogilvie, B. M., and McLaren, D. J., The immune mechanism which expels the intestinal stage of *Trichenella spiralis, Immunology,* 30, 7, 1976.
72. Gabriel, B. W. and Justus, D. E., Quantitation of immediate and delayed hypersensitivity responses in *Trichinella*-infected mice, *Int. Arch. Allergy Appl. Immunol.*, 60, 275, 1979.
73. Jacqueline, E., Vernes, A., Bout, D., and Biguet, J., *Trichinella spiralis:* facteurs immuntaires inhibiteurs de la production de larves. II. Premièreanalyse *in vitro* des facteurs humoraux et sécrétoires actifs chez les souris, le rat, et la miniporc infestés ou immunisés, *Exp. Parasitol.*, 45, 42, 1978.
74. Taliaferro, W. H. and Sarles, M. P., The cellular reactions in the skin, lungs and intestine of normal and immune rats after infection with *Nippostrongylus muris, J. Infect.Dis.*, 54, 157, 1939.
75. Jones, V. E., Edwards, A. J., and Ogilvie, B. M., The circulating immunoglobulins involved in protective immunity to the intestinal stage of *Nippostrongylus brasiliensis* in the rat, *Immunology,* 18, 621, 1970.
76. Nawa, Y., Parish, C. R., and Miller, H. R. P., The protective capacities of fractionated immune thoracic duct lymphocytes against *Nippostrongylus brasiliensis, Cell. Immunol.*, 37, 41, 1978.
77. Poulain, J., Luffau, G., and Pery, P., *Nippostrongylus brasiliensis* in the rat. Immune response in serum and intestinal secretions, *Ann. Immunol.*, 127, 215, 1976.
78. Sinski, E. and Holmes, P. H., *Nippostrongylus brasiliensis:* systemic and local immune response in parasitized rats, *Exp. Parasitol.*, 43, 382, 1977.
79. Woodbury, R. G., Miller, H. R. P., Huntley, J. F., Newlands, G. F. J., Palliser, A. C., and Wakelin, D., Mucosal mast cells are functionally active during the spontaneous expulsion of primary intestinal nematode infections in the rat, *Nature,* 312, 450, 1984.
80. Lee, G. B. and Ogilvie, B. M., The mucus layer in intestinal nematode infections, in *The Mucosal Immune System in Health and Disease,* Ogra, P. and Bienenstock, J., Eds., Ross Laboratories, Columbus, Ohio, 1981, 175.
81. Miller, H. R. P., Huntley, J. F., and Wallace, G. R., Immune exclusion and mucus trapping during the rapid expulsion of *Nippostrongylus brasiliensis* from primed rats, *Immunology,* 44, 419, 1981.
82. Castro, G. A., Hessel, J. J., and Whalen, G., Altered intestinal fluid movement in responses to *Trichinella spiralis* in immunized rats, *Parasite Immunol.*, 1, 259, 1979.
83. Castro, G. A. and Harari, Y, Intestinal epithelial membrane changes in rats immune to *Trichinella spiralis, Mol. Biochem. Parasitol.*, 6, 191, 1982.
84. Bell, R. G. and McGregor, D. D., Requirement for two discrete stimuli for induction of the intestinal rapid expulsion response against *Trichinella spiralis* in rats, *Infect. Immun.*, 29, 186, 1980.
85. Ehrenford, F. A., The life cycle of *Nematospiroides dubius* Baylis (Nematoda: Heligosomoidae), *J. Parasitol.*, 40, 480, 1954.
86. Pritchard, D. I., Williams, D. J. L., Behnke, J. M., and Lee, T. D. G., The role of the IgG_1 hypergammaglobulinaemia in immunity to the gastrointestinal nematode *Nematospiroides dubius.* The immunochemical purification, antigen specificity and *in vivo* anti-parasite effect of IgG_1 from immune serum, *Immunology,* 43, 353, 1983.

87. Pritchard, D. I., Behnke, J. M., and Williams, D. J. L., Primary infection sera and IgG_1 do not block host protective immunity to *Nematospiroides dubius*, *Immunology*, 51, 73, 1984.
88. Rose, M. E. and Hesketh, P., Immunity to coccidiosis: T-lymphocyte- or B-lymphocyte-deficient animals, *Infect. Immun.*, 26, 630, 1979.
89. Rose, M. E. and Hesketh, P., Immunity to coccidia in chickens: adoptive transfer with peripheral blood lymphocytes and spleen cells, *Parasite Immunol.*, 54, 171, 1982.
90. Davis, P. J., Parry, S. H., and Porter, P., The role of secretory IgA in anti-coccidial immunity in the chicken, *Immunology*, 34, 879, 1978.
91. Davis, P. J. and Porter, P., A mechanism for secretory IgA-mediated inhibition of the cell penetration and intracellular development of *Eimeria tenella*, *Immunology*, 36, 471, 1979.
92. Patton, W. H., *In vitro* phagocytosis of coccidia by macrophages from the blood of infected chickens, *J. Parasitol.*, 56, 260, 1970.
93. Rose, M. E. and Lee, D. L., Interactions *in vitro* between sporozoites of *Eimeria tenella* and host peritoneal exudate cells: electron microscopical observations, *Z. Parasitenkd.*, 54, 1, 1977.
94. Millard, B. J. and Lawn, A. M., Parasite-host relationships during the development of *Eimeria dispersa* Tyzzer 1929, in the turkey *(Meleagris gallopavo gallopavo)* with a description of intestinal intraepithelial leucocytes, *Parasitology*, 84, 13, 1982.
95. Rose, M. E., Ogilvie, B. M., and Bradley, J. W. A., Intestinal mast cell response in rats and chickens to coccidiosis, with some properties of chicken mast cells, *Int. Arch. Allergy Appl. Immunol.*, 63, 21, 1980.
96. Rose, M. E., Hesketh, P., and Ogilvie, B. M., Peripheral blood leucocyte response to coccidial infection: a comparison of the response in rats and chickens and its correlation with resistance to reinfection, *Immunology*, 36, 71, 1979.
97. Stoll, N., The occurrence of self-cure and protection in typical nematode parasitism, *J. Parasitol.*, 15, 147, 1928.
98. Stewart, D. F., "Self-cure" in nematode infestations of sheep, *Nature*, 176, 1273, 1955.
99. Smith, W. D., Jackson, F., Jackson, E., Williams, J., Willadsen, S. N., and Fehilly, G. B., Resistance to *Haemonchus contortus* transferred between genetically histocompatible sheep with immune lymphocytes, *Res. Vet. Sci.*, 37, 199, 1984.
100. Adams, D. B. and Rothwell, T. L. N., *Trichostrongylus colubriformis:* host factors influencing the transfer of immunity in guinea pigs using mesenteric lymph node cells, *Exp. Parasitol.*, 42, 121, 1977.
101. Smith, W. D., Anti-larval antibodies in the serum and abomasal mucus of sheep hyperinfected with *Haemonchus contortus*, *Res. Vet. Sci.*, 22, 334, 1977.
102. Cripps, A. W. and Rothwell, T. L. W., Immune responses of sheep to the parasitic nematode *Trichostrongylus colubriformis:* infections in Thiry-vella loops, *Aust. J. Exp. Biol. Med. Sci.*, 56, 99, 1978.
103. Cripps, A. W. and Adams, D. B., Flow and protein composition of intestinal lymph in sheep infected with the enteric nematode *Trichostrongylus colubriformis*, *Aust. J. Exp. Biol. Med.Sci.*, 56, 225, 1978.
104. Smith, W. D., Jackson, F., Jackson, E., Williams, J., and Miller, H. R. P., Manifestations of resistance to ovine ostertagiasis associated with immunological responses in the gastric lymph, *J. Comp. Pathol.*, 94, 591, 1984.
105. Smith, W. D., Jackson, F., Jackson, E., Dawson, A. M., and Burrells, C., Changes in the flow and composition of gastric lymph in sheep repeatedly infected with *Ostertagia circumcincta*, *J. Comp. Pathol.*, 91, 553, 1981.
106. Jackson, F., Angus, K. W., and Coop, R. L., The development of morphological changes in the small intestine of lambs continuously infected with *Trichostrongylus vitrinus*, *Res. Vet. Sci.*, 34, 301, 1983.
107. Dobson, C., Changes in the protein content of the serum and intestinal mucus of sheep with reference to the histology of the gut and immunological response to *Oesophagostomum columbianum* infections, *Parasitology*, 57, 201, 1967.
108. Dobson, C. and Bawden, R. J., Studies on the immunity of sheep to *Oesophagostomum columbianum*. Effects of low-protein diet on resistance to infection and cellular reactions in the gut, *Parasitology*, 69, 239, 1974.
109. Christie, M. G., Hart, R., Angus, K. W., Devoy, J., and Patterson, J. E., Resistance to *Haemonchus contortus* in sheep given repeated daily doses of 10,000 infective larvae, *J. Comp. Pathol.*, 88, 157, 1978.
110. Dobson, C., Studies on the immunity of sheep to *Oesophagostomum columbianum:* proteins and haemagglutinating antibodies in mucous exudates and intestinal tissue extracts, *Aust. J. Agric. Res.*, 17, 779, 1966.
111. Murray, M., Miller, H. R. P., and Jarrett, W. F. H., The globule leukocyte and its derivation from the subepithelial mast cell, *Lab. Invest.*, 19, 222, 1968.

112. Huntley, J. F., Newlands, G., and Miller, H. R. P., The isolation and characterization of globule leukocytes: their derivation from mucosal mast cells in parasitized sheep, *Parasite Immunol.*, 6, 371, 1984.
113. Stewart, D. F., Studies on resistance of sheep to infestation with *Haemonchus contortus* and *Trichostrongylus* spp. and on the immunological reactions of sheep exposed to infestation, *Aust. J. Agric. Res.*, 4, 100, 1953.
114. Armour, J., Jarrett, W. F. H., and Jennings, F. N., Experimental *Ostertagia circumcincta* infections in sheep: development and pathogenesis of a single infection, *Am. J. Vet. Res.*, 27, 1267, 1966.
115. Dineen, J. K., Gregg, P., and Lascelles, A. K., The response of lambs to vaccination at weaning with irradiated *Trichostrongylus colubriformis* larvae: segregation into "responders" and "non responders", *Int. J. Parasitol.*, 8, 59, 1978.
116. Dineen, J. K. and Windon, R. G., The effect of sire selection on the response of lambs to vaccination with irradiated *Trichostrongylus colubriformis* larvae, *Int. J. Parasitol.*, 10, 189, 1980.
117. Cohen, S. and Warren, K. S., Eds., *Immunology of Parasitic Infections*, Blackwell Scientific, Oxford, 1982.
118. Ament, M. E. and Rubin, C. E., Relation of giardiasis to abnormal intestinal structure and function in gastrointestinal immunodeficiency syndromes, *Gastroenterology*, 62, 216, 1972.
119. Halstead, S. B. and Sadun, E. H., Alimentary hypersensitivity induced by *Giardia lamblia*. Report of a case of acute meat intolerance, *Ann. Intern. Med.*, 62, 561, 1965.
120. Rendtorff, R. C., The experimental transmission of human intestinal protozoan parasites. II. *Giardia lamblia* cysts given in capsules, *Am. J. Hyg.*, 59, 209, 1954.
121. Rendtorff, R. C. and Holt, C. J., The experimental transmission of human intestinal protozoan parasites. IV. Attempts to transmit *Entamoeba coli* and *Giardia lamblia* cysts by water, *Am. J. Hyg.*, 60, 327, 1954.
122. Grove, D. I., Immunity in human helminth infections, in *Biology and Control of Endoparasites*, Symons, L. E. A., Donald, A. D., and Dineen, J. K., Eds., Academic Press, New York, 1982, 375.
123. Ogilvie, B. M. and De Savigny, D., Immune response to nematodes, in *Immunology of Parasitic Infections*, Cohen, S. and Warren, K. S., Eds., Blackwell Scientific, Oxford, 1982, 715.
124. O'Donnell, I. J. and Mitchell, G. F., An investigation of the antigens of *Ascaris lumbrocoides* using a radio immunoassay and sera of naturally infected humans, *Int. Arch. Allergy Appl. Immunol.*, 61, 213, 1980.
125. Miller, H. R. P., The origin, structure and function of mucosal mast cells, a brief review, *Biol. Cell.*, 39, 229, 1980.
126. Filho, E. C., Strongyloidiasis, in *Clinics in Gastroenterology*, Vol. 7, No. 1, W. B. Saunders, Philadelphia, 1978, 179.
127. Moqbel, R., Histopathological changes following primary, secondary and repeated infections of rats with *Strongyloides ratti*, with special reference to tissue eosinophils, *Parasite Immunol.*, 2, 11, 1980.
128. Jarrett, E. E. E. and Miller, H. R. P., Production and activities of IgE in helminth infection, *Prog. Allergy*, 31, 178, 1982.
129. Dessein, A. J., Parker, N. L., James, S. L., and David, J. R., IgE antibody and resistance to infection. I. Selective suppression of the IgE antibody response in rats diminishes the resistance and the eosinophil response to *Trichinella spiralis* infection, *J. Exp. Med.*, 153, 423, 1981.
130. Pery, P. and Luffau, G., Antigens of helminths, in *The Antigens, Vol. 5, Sela, M., Ed.*, Academic Press, New York, 1979, 83.
131. Ogilvie, B. M. and Jones, V. E., Reaginic antibodies and immunity to *Nippostrongylus brasiliensis* in the rat. I. The effect of thymectomy, neonatal infections and splenectomy, *Parasitology*, 57, 335, 1967.
132. Jarrett, E. E. E. and Ferguson, A., Effect of T cell depletion on the potentiated reagin response, *Nature (London)*, 250, 420, 1974.
133. Suemara, M. and Ishizaka, K., Potentiation of IgE response *in vitro* by T cells from rats infected with *Nippostrongylus brasiliensis*, *J. Immunol.*, 123, 918, 1979.
134. Hirashima, M., Yodoi, J., and Ishizaka, K., Regulatory role of IgE binding factors from rat T lymphocytes, III. IgE specific suppressive factor with IgE binding activity, *J. Immunol.*, 125, 1442, 1980.
135. Urban, J. F., Ishizaka, T., and Ishizaka, K., IgE B cell-generating factor from lymph node cells of rats infected with *Nippostrongylus brasiliensis*. I. Source of IgE-bearing cells in neonatally thymectomized animals, *J. Immunol.*, 118, 1982, 1978.
136. Urban, J. F. and Ishizaka, K., IgE B cell-generating factor from lymph node cells of rats infected with *Nippostrongylus brasiliensis*. II. Effector mechanisms of IgE B cell generating factor, *J. Immunol.*, 121, 199, 1978.
137. Ruitenberg, E. J. and Elgersma, A., Absence of intestinal mast cell response in congenitally athymic mice during *Trichinella spiralis* infection, *Nature*, 264, 258, 1976.

138. Befus, A. D., Pearce, F. L., Gauldie, J., Horsewood, P., and Bienenstock, J., Mucosal mast cells. I. Isolation and functional characteristics of rat intestinal mast cells, *J. Immunol.*, 128, 2475, 1982.
139. Pearce, F. L., Befus, A. D., Gauldie, J., and Bienenstock, J., Mucosal mast cells. II. Effects of anti-allergic compounds on histamine secretion by isolated intestinal mast cells, *J. Immunol.*, 128, 2481, 1982.
140. Alizadeh, H. and Wakelin, D., Genetic factors controlling the intestinal mast cell response in mice infected with *Trichinella spiralis*, *Clin. Exp. Immunol.*, 49, 331, 1982.
141. Haig, D. M., McKee, T. A., Jarrett, E. E. E., Woodbury, R. G., and Miller, H. R. P., Generation of mucosal mast cells is stimulated *in vitro* by factors derived from T cells of helminth-infected rats, *Nature*, 300, 188, 1982.
142. Guy-Grand, D., Dy, M., Luffau, G., and Vassalli, P., Gut mucosal mast cells. Origin, traffic and differentiation, *J. Exp. Med.*, 160, 12, 1984.
143. Mayrhofer, G., Bazin, M., and Gowans, J. L., Nature of cells binding anti-IgE in rats immunized with *Nippostrongylus brasiliensis*: IgE synthesis in regional nodes and concentration in mucosal mast cells, *Eur. J. Immunol.*, 13, 112, 1976.
144. Despommier, D., Weisbroth, S., and Fass, C., Circulating eosinophils and trichinosis in the rat: the parasitic stage responsible for induction during infection, *J. Parasitol.*, 60, 280, 1974.
145. Prowse, S. J., Ey, P. L., and Jenkin, C. R., Immunity to *Nematospiroides dubius*: cell and immunoglobulin changes and the onset of immunity in mice, *Aust. J. Exp. Biol. Med. Sci.*, 56, 237, 1978.
146. Rothwell, T. L. W., Studies of the responses of basophil and eosinophil leucocytes and mast cells to the nematode *Trichostrongylus colubriformis*. I. Observations during the expulsion of first and second infections by guinea-pigs. *J. Pathol.*, 116, 51, 1975.
147. Ruitenberg, E. J., Elgersma, A., Kruizinga, W., and Leenstra, F., *Trichinella spiralis* infection in congenitally athymic (nude) mice. Parasitological, serological and haematological studies with observations on intestinal pathology, *Immunology*, 33, 581, 1977.
148. Gleich, G. J., Olson, G. M., and Herlich, H., The effect of antiserum to eosinophils on susceptibility and acquired immunity of the guinea pig to *Trichostrongylus colubriformis*, *Immunology*, 37, 873, 1979.
149. Spry, C. J. F., Eosinophilia and hypereosinophilic syndromes, *Trans. R. Soc. Trop. Med. Hyg.*, 74 (Suppl.), 3, 1980.
150. Vadas, M. A., Genetic control of eosinophilia in mice. Genes expressed in bone marrow-derived cells control high responsiveness, *J. Immunol.*, 128, 691, 1982.
151. Wakelin, D. and Donachie, A. M., Genetic control of eosinophilia. Mouse strain variation in response to antigens of parasite origin, *Clin. Exp. Immunol.*, 51, 239, 1983.
152. Chase, M. W., Inhibition of experimental drug allergy by prior feeding of the sensitizing agent, *Proc. Soc. Exp. Biol. Med.*, 61, 257, 1946.
153. Miller, S. D. and Hanson, D. G., Inhibition of specific immune responses by feeding protein antigens. IV. Evidence for tolerance and specific active suppression of cell-mediated immune responses to ovalbumin, *J. Immunol.*, 123, 2344, 1979.
154. Mattingly, J. A. and Waksman, B. H., Immunological suppression after oral administration of antigen. I. Specific suppressor cells formed in rat Peyer's patches after oral administration of sheep erythrocytes and their systemic migration, *J. Immunol.*, 121, 1878, 1979.
155. Faubert, G. M., Depression of the plaque-forming cells to sheep red blood cells by the newborn larvae of *Trichinella spiralis*, *Immunology*, 30, 485, 1976.
156. Faubert, G. and Tanner, C. E., *Trichinella spiralis*: inhibition of sheep haemagglutinins in mice, *Exp. Parasitol.*, 30, 120, 1971.
157. Haig, D. M., Lima, G. C., and Mota, I., Antibody suppression in mice infected with *Nippostrongylus brasiliensis*, *Parasite Immunol.*, 2, 175, 1980.
158. Duszynski, D. W., Russell, D., Roy, S. A., and Castro, G. A., Suppressed rejection of *Trichinella spiralis* in immunized rats concurrently infected with *Eimeria nieschulzi*, *J. Parasitol.*, 64, 83, 1978.
159. Ali, N. M. H. and Behnke, J. M., Non specific immunodepression by larval and adult *Nematospiroides dubius*, *Parasitology*, 88, 153, 1983.
160. Pritchard, D. I., Ali, N. M. H., and Behnke, J. M., Analysis of the mechanism of immunodepression following heterologous antigenic stimulation during concurrent infection with *Nematospiroides dubius*, *Immunoloy*, 51, 633, 1984.
161. Behnke, J. M., Hannah, J., and Pritchard, D. I., Evidence that adult *Nematospiroides dubius* impair the immune response of mice to a challenge infection, *Parasite Immunol.*, 5, 397, 1983.
162. Hagan, P. and Wakelin, D., *Nematospiroides dibius*: effect of infection on lymphocyte responses to *Trichinella spiralis* in mice, *Exp. Parasitol*, 54, 157, 1982.
163. Wassom, D. L., Dougherty, D. A., Krco, C. J., and David, C. S., H-2-Controlled, dose dependent suppression of the response which expels adult *Trichinella spiralis* from the small intestine of mice, *Immunology*, 51, 625, 1984.

164. Grencis, R. K. and Wakelin, D., Immunity to *Trichinella spiralis* in mice. Factors involved in direct anti-worm effects, *Wiad. Parazytol.*, 29, 387, 1983.
165. Grencis, R. K., Crawford, C. C., Pritchard, D. I., Behnke, J. M., and Wakelin, D., Immunization of mice with surface antigens from the muscle larvae of *Trichinella spiralis* parasite, *Immunology,* in press.

Chapter 5

IMMUNE RESPONSES IN CHRONIC GASTROINTESTINAL DISEASES

Nigel Mike and Peter Asquith

TABLE OF CONTENTS

I. Introduction 26

II. Gastritis 26
A. Type A Chronic Atrophic Gastritis and Pernicious Anemia 27
1. Humoral Immunity 28
a. Gastric Antibodies 28
b. Intrinsic Factor Antibody 28
c. Parietal Cell Antibody 29
2. Cellular Immunity 29
3. Immunopathogenesis of Pernicious Anemia 30
B. Type B Atrophic Gastritis 32
C. Varioliform Gastritis 32
D. Eosinophilic Gastroenteritis 33

III. Celiac Disease 34
A. Humoral Immunity 35
B. Cell-Mediated Immunity 36
1. Lymphocyte Studies 36
C. Jejunal Mucosa 37
D. Skin Testing 37
E. Genetic Studies 38
F. Immune Pathogenesis of Celiac Disease 39

IV. CMPI 40
A. Clinical Features 41
B. Immunology of CMPI 42
1. Type I 42
2. Type III 42
3. Type IV 43

V. Soya Protein Enteropathy 43
A. Pathogenesis of Soya Protein Enteropathy 44
B. Soya Protein Hypersensitivity in Celiac Disease 44

VI. Inflammatory Bowel Disease 45
A. Crohn's Disease 45
1. Immunological Etiology 45
2. The Mucosal Lesion 47
3. Macrophages and Neutrophils 48
4. Humoral Responses 49
5. Cell-Mediated Immunity 49
6. Other Factors in the Pathogenesis of Crohn's Disease 50
a. Infection 50

b. Diet 50
c. Smoking 51
B. Ulcerative Colitis 51
1. Immunological Etiology 51
2. The Mucosal Lesion 52
3. Macrophages 52
4. Humoral Responses 52
5. Cell-Mediated Immunity 53
6. Other Factors in the Pathogenesis of Ulcerative Colitis 53
a. Infection 53
b. Diet 54
c. Smoking 54
C. The Pathogenesis of Inflammatory Bowel Disease 54

VII. Conclusions 55

References 55

I. INTRODUCTION

There seems to be little doubt that immunological mechanisms play a role of varying significance in several important gastrointestinal syndromes. However, it is less clear whether such reactions are primary events and hence can be regarded as the basic cause of the disease(s). Research aimed at answering this question has often been severely compromised because the nature of the immunizing antigen is unknown; for example, in Crohn's disease and ulcerative colitis a number of agents have been considered, varying from foodstuffs to infectious organisms. Exceptionally, the "antigen" has been partially identified, such as gluten in celiac disease. However, even in such favorable experimental situations as celiac disease, we still do not know whether the immunological events are just secondary phenomena.

This chapter presents some of the evidence for the immunopathogenic basis for gastritis, celiac disease, cows milk protein intolerance CMPI, soya protein enteropathy, Crohn's disease, and ulcerative colitis; the clinical features of each of these conditions are only briefly considered.

II. GASTRITIS

The diagnosis of gastritis depends on serological, secretory, endoscopic, and histological findings, and using these criteria, it is classified into five types (Table 1). Of these, hypertrophic gastritis has no immunological basis and is not further considered.

Acute gastritis is manifested by necrosis of the surface mucosa, with hyperemia, edema, and hemorrhage. Precipitants include drugs, such as aspirin and other nonsteroidal anti-inflammatory agents, alcohol, and chemicals such as bile, strong acids and alkalis, and gold. Major stress, occurring in burns, head injury, renal failure, and radiation, has also been implicated, while angioneurotic edema and urticaria are rarer causes.

Chronic gastritis may be superficial or atrophic. Chronic superficial gastritis is rather similar to acute gastritis, with probably the same precipitating factors, in particular alcohol, tobacco, and nonsteroidal anti-inflammatory drugs. Lymphocytes and

Table 1
CLASSIFICATION OF GASTRITIS

Acute gastritis
Chronic gastritis
  Superficial
  Atrophic: types A and B
Hypertrophic gastritis (ménétrier's)
Varioliform (verrucous) gastritis
Eosinophilic gastritis

Table 2
CHRONIC ATROPHIC GASTRITIS

Site of disease	Type A Fundus and body	Type B Antrum
Occurrence	25%	75%
Symptoms	No	Common
Peptic ulcer	−	+
Pernicious anemia	+	−
Carcinoma	+	+
Associated autoimmune endocrinopathies	+	−
Intrinsic factor antibodies	++	−
Parietal cell antibodies	+++	±
Gastrin antibodies	−	+
G cell mass	↑	↓
Serum gastrin	↑	N
Acid output	Achlorhydria	Reduced
Pepsinogen I	↓↓	↓
Pepsinogen II	N	↑

plasma cells infiltrate the lamina propria between the gastric pits, but the glandular structure is normal.

Chronic atrophic gastritis on the other hand is a progressive disease, culminating in complete loss of the gastric glands, mucosal thinning, and gastric atrophy. The lamina propria is infiltrated with plasma cells and lymphocytes, whereas the gastric pits are shortened with a reduction in the number of parietal and chief cells. Intestinal metaplasia is common, with the gastric body mucosa being replaced by antral or small intestinal type mucosa. Chronic atrophic gastritis has been further subdivided into types A and B by Strickland and Mackay[1] (Table 2). Type A, or autoimmune gastritis, affects the gastric fundus and body, with only mild inflammation of the antrum, whereas, type B gastritis principally affects the antrum.[2] Gastric autoantibodies, achlorhydria, and pernicious anemia are found in type A gastritis.

A. Type A Chronic Atrophic Gastritis and Pernicious Anemia

The incidence of atrophic gastritis increases with age; indeed, it may be part of the aging process.[1] Organ-specific autoimmune diseases, in particular Hashimoto's thyroiditis, thyrotoxicosis, and myxedema, are frequently associated with pernicious anemia.[3] Thus Carmel and Spencer[4] found that 48% of 162 patients with pernicious anemia had clinical or subclinical thyroid disease.[49] Furthermore, insulin-dependent diabetes mellitus, Addison's disease idiopathic hypoparathyroidism, and vitiligo and much less commonly the sicca syndrome, dermatitis herpetiformis, and myasthenia

Table 3
THE FREQUENCY (%) OF GASTRIC AND THYROID AUTOANTIBODIES[a]

Patient group	Parietal cell antibody	Intrinsic factor antibody	Thyroglobulin antibody	Thyroid microsomal antibody
Healthy subjects	5—16	0	0—15	NA
Pernicious anemia	75—88	38—70	34.6	52.5
Thyroid disease	25—40	0—5	100	97.8
Addison's disease	12—40	20	NA	NA
Insulin-dependent diabetes mellitus	21—28	3—4	NA	NA
Hypoparathyroidism	16	NA	NA	NA
Iron-deficiency anemia	17—20	NA	NA	NA

[a] NA = data not available.

gravis are also found. Patients with pernicious anemia have an increased incidence of tissue antibodies as shown in Table 3,[5-7] with thyroid antibodies occurring in up to 50% of patients. Conversely, gastric parietal cell antibodies are found in from 12 to 40% of patients with other autoimmune diseases but who do not have pernicious anemia. Nevertheless, intrinsic factor antibody is relatively specific for pernicious anemia.[8]

Genetic studies have shown that pernicious anemia and atrophic gastritis are familial diseases. Thus 20% of relatives of patients with pernicious anemia have or are liable to develop the disease.[8] Gastric parietal cell antibodies are also common (20 to 30%) in such relatives. Blood group A is strongly associated with pernicious anemia, whereas the HLA antigens, A3, A10, and B7 are only weakly related.[9-11] The HLA-DR2 and HLA-DR5 antigens are also increased with a relative risk of pernicious anemia of 5.93.[7,12,13] Thomsen and co-workers[14] and Feldt-Rasmussen and co-workers[7] also found that DR2 patients frequently possessed intrinsic factor antibodies, whereas DR5 patients did not. Interestingly, a similar histocompatibility profile (increased HLA-DR2 and DR5 and decreased DR3) is found in Hashimoto's thyroiditis[7,12] in contradistinction to the other organ-specific autoimmune diseases in which there is an increase in HLA-DR3.

1. Humoral Immunity

a. Gastric Antibodies

In pernicious anemia, antibodies are found to two antigenic components of the gastric parietal cell. One is intrinsic factor, a glycoprotein of 60,000 mol wt, which is situated peripherally within the cell. This is essential for the absorption of vitamin B_{12}, and its secretion is reduced in direct proportion to the degree of gastric mucosal damage.[15] The second is an insoluble lipoprotein of the microvilli of the parietal cell secretory canalicular system.

b. Intrinsic Factor Antibody

Two distinct types of intrinsic factor antibodies have been described in pernicious anemia. Type I is a blocking antibody which attaches to the binding site for vitamin B_{12} on the intrinsic factor and therefore prevents free vitamin B_{12} from binding to the intrinsic factor.[16] In contrast, type II is a binding antibody which can attach to the free intrinsic factor or the intrinsic factor-B_{12} complex.

Type I antibody is found in approximately 70% of patients, whereas type II is found in 35 to 40%[17] and is very rarely found in the absence of type I antibody. In animal studies, immunization with human intrinsic factor elicits a type I antibody response, whereas immunization with intrinsic factor-B_{12} complex results in a type II response; the addition of B_{12} also produced higher levels of type I antibody.[16] Human intrinsic factor serum antibodies are mainly of immunoglobulin G (IgG) class, with a small amount of IgA and rarely IgM.[18] They are found more frequently in gastric juice than serum, sometimes in the absence of serum antibody; juice antibodies may be either IgG or IgA[18] or even secretory IgA (SIgA) class.[19] Finally, lamina propria plasma cells have been shown to produce type II antibody.

c. Parietal Cell Antibody

Antibodies to the parietal cell canaliculus are found in up to 90% of patients with pernicious anemia. It is also found in patients with gastritis but who do not have pernicious anemia. Its incidence also increases with age, 2% of healthy subjects under 20 years of age in contrast to 16% of those over 60. The antibody is also found in gastric juice, though less frequently than in serum,[18] and it is more likely to be of IgA class, whereas serum antibody is usually IgG.

Parietal cell antibody reacts with an antigen situated in the microsomal fraction of the cell within the membranes of the microvilli of the secretory canaliculi.[20] Furthermore, in 1980 Masala and co-workers,[21] using immunofluorescent techniques, showed that serum from patients with pernicious anemia containing parietal cell canalicular antibody reacted in vitro with the surface membranes of parietal cells. De Aizpura[22] later confirmed this finding and suggested that this parietal cell surface antibody reacts with antigenic determinants that are probably different from the microsomal antigen recognized by parietal cell cytoplasmic antibody.

In a further study, De Aizpura and co-workers[23] showed that serum from patients with pernicious anemia was strongly cytotoxic to parietal cell-enriched gastric mucosal cells. This cytotoxic activity correlated with the presence of the parietal cell surface membrane autoantibody[24] and was not related to the presence or absence of parietal cell cytoplasmic antibody or intrinsic factor antibody. The cytotoxic activity was also unrelated to the patient's age or ABO group.

2. Cellular Immunity

There is conflicting evidence on the role of cell-mediated immunity in pernicious anemia. In two studies, lymphocyte blast transformation occurred in a number of such patients when their lymphocytes were incubated in vitro with gastric juice or intrinsic factor,[25,26] but transformation did not occur in another report.[27] Using the leukocyte migration inhibition test, cell-mediated immunity to intrinsic factor has been observed.[26,28,29] Unfortunately, purified intrinsic factor was not used, and Finlayson et al.[30] in 1972 demonstrated cellular hypersensitivity to antigens in gastric juice which were not B_{12} binding, casting doubt on the specificity and relevance of the previous studies. Other gastric antigens such as gastric mitochondria and microsomes and liver mitochondria can also elicit a cell-mediated response.[31] Overall these authors and others could find no correlation between the humoral response with intrinsic factor and parietal cell canalicular antibody and the cellular response to intrinsic factor or gastric microsomes.

In a recent study by Kountouras and colleagues,[32] three of ten patients with type A atrophic gastritis showed significant inhibition of leukocyte migration on exposure to a crude gastric mucosal antigen, and four of the ten showed inhibition with hog intrinsic factor. In this study the degree of migration inhibition also correlated with the severity of the mucosal atrophy, and on this basis it was suggested that cell-mediated immunity accounts for the severity of the mucosal damage. However, as with previous studies, the impurity of the antigens makes this report difficult to interpret. Concerning nonspecific cellular hypersensitivity, as assessed by lymphocyte counts, delayed hypersensitivity skin responses, and phytohemagglutinin-induced blastogenesis, this appears normal in patients with pernicious anemia[33] irrespective of treatment status.[34] However, in the latter study, of seven patients who had negative skin responses to tuberculin prior to treatment, five developed cutaneous hypersensitivity after vitamin B_{12}.

3. Immunopathogenesis of Pernicious Anemia

The evidence that immune mechanisms are etiologically significant in pernicious anemia is both indirect and direct. A suggestive indirect feature is the invariable infiltration of the lamina propria of the stomach. Also, as previously mentioned, pernicious anemia clusters with other organ-specific autoimmune diseases such as thyroid disease, Addison's disease, and insulin-dependent diabetes mellitus.

The observations with respect to gastric autoantibodies provides the most convincing direct evidence. Intrinsic factor antibody is relatively specific for pernicious anemia and rarely occurs otherwise. The parietal cell canalicular antibody is nearly always found in the presence of gastritis, though uncommonly in type B gastritis.[35] These autoantibodies are not found in patients with gastric ulcer, carcinoma, or biliary gastritis; they are likely to be related to etiology of pernicious anemia, rather than being secondary to mucosal damage On the other hand, pernicious anemia does occur in some patients who do not have serum or gastric juice intrinsic factor or gastric parietal cell antibodies. These latter patients may have a cell-mediated immune response, or alternatively the damage may be due to the parietal cell surface autoantibody described by Masala et al.[21] and De Aizpura et al.[22] Furthermore, pernicious anemia also occurs in patients with panhypogammaglobulinemia,[36] and in these individuals, serum gastric autoantibodies are also absent. These patients, however, also differ in other respects from patients with classical pernicious anemia, and it is possible that other nonimmunological mechanisms account for their atrophic gastritis.

Further direct evidence that these gastric autoantibodies are of major importance in the pathogenesis of pernicious anemia is provided by several studies. Rose and Chanarin[37] demonstrated that type I intrinsic factor antibody can be completely complexed with intrinsic factor in the gastric juice. They subsequently showed that the amount of vitamin B_{12} absorption was related to the presence and origin of intrinsic factor antibody.[38]

Vitamin B_{12} absorption was impaired when intrinsic factor was present in serum but not in gastric juice, more impaired if intrinsic factor antibody was present in gastric juice but not in the serum, and maximally impaired when the antibody was present in both juice and serum. It was postulated that this combination of impaired B_{12} absorption and complexing of the available remaining intrinsic factor could eventually cause pernicious anemia.

It is therefore probable that intrinsic factor antibody is involved directly in the malabsorption of vitamin B_{12}. Whether it also causes atrophic gastritis is less clear. Animal studies have shown that when rats are repeatedly injected with human serum intrinsic factor antibody, they slowly develop atrophy of the chief cells in the gastric mucosa, cells which produce rat intrinsic factor.[39] Interestingly, there was no inflammatory response. Likewise, there have been reports of humans who have intrinsic factor antibody without pernicious anemia. However, these patients do have atrophic gastritis, and it may be that in time they will develop vitamin B_{12} deficiency.

Concerning gastric parietal cell antibody, it now seems likely that it is of prime importance in the development of gastric mucosal damage. Early animal studies suggested this possibility. Hausamen and co-workers[40] demonstrated in vitro that human gastric parietal cell antibody inhibited acid production by bullfrog gastric mucosa. They subsequently also showed that reexposure of injected guinea pig gastric parietal cell antibody resulted in an acute inflammatory reaction within the gastric mucosa.[41]

In 1980, Masala et al.[21] reported that serum from patients with pernicious anemia containing parietal cell antibody reacted with the surface membranes of parietal cells. At the same time, Loveridge et al.[42] found that these antibodies could inhibit parietal cell function. De Aizpura and colleagues[22] showed that the parietal cell surface-reactive autoantibody reacted with different autoantigenic determinants to the canalicular autoantibody. They subsequently showed that this surface-reactive autoantibody was cytotoxic to gastric mucosal cells and that the cytotoxic factor resided in the IgG fraction. Complement was also required for cell lysis. (The parietal cell canalicular antibody and intrinsic factor antibody were not cytotoxic in this test system. In this respect, previous studies had suggested that the parietal cell antibody might be complement fixing and that this was the mode of its toxicity. Thus Jacob and Glass[43] reported that patients with pernicious anemia had significantly lower complement levels, whereas Te Velde[44] demonstrated complement fixation on parietal cells of rodent stomach exposed to parietal cell antibody. It seems likely therefore that the complement-fixing autoantibody to parietal cell surfaces is the cause of loss of parietal cells in pernicious anemia. Supportive evidence for this comes from the work of Tanaka and Glass[45] who repeatedly injected human IgG parietal cell antibody into rats. Over a period of weeks there was a reduction in parietal cell mass with a concomitant reduction in gastric acid output.

In summary it appears that intrinsic factor antibody impairs the absorption of vitamin B_{12}, whereas gastric parietal cell antibody causes loss of parietal cells and achlorhydria. Further support for an antibody-dependent immune basis to pernicious anemia comes from the work of Kaye and co-workers,[46] who studied lymphocyte subpopulations in the gastric mucosa of patients with pernicious anemia. Using monoclonal antibodies, they found the concentrations of T, T helper (T_h), T suppressor (T_s), and non-T cells were significantly increased in patients with pernicious anemia. The most striking increase (sixfold) was in the non-T cells, most of which were presumed to be B cells. This was quite different from the findings in patients with gastritis associated with peptic ulceration and was considered further evidence that the mucosal damage in pernicious anemia was mediated by humoral mechanisms.

The data of cellular mechanisms should, however, not be dismissed with respect to the pathogenesis of atrophic gastritis. In those pernicious anemia patients without autoantibodies and in those with panhypogammaglobulinemia, it is assumed that the atrophic gastritis is caused by cell-mediated immune mechanisms. A number of studies have shown that lymphocytes of some patients with pernicious anemia can undergo blast, transformation or produce lymphokine in the presence of gastric antigens. Early studies in pernicious anemia[47] also showed that steroids caused regeneration of gastric parietal cells and structural improvement. They also caused increased intrinsic factor secretion with improved vitamin B_{12} absorption. As steroids are thought to act predominantly on T cells, this was considered further evidence of the importance of delayed hypersensitivity in pernicious anemia.

Further cellular evidence is provided by animal studies. Rhesus monkeys repeatedly injected with gastric antigens developed cutaneous delayed hypersensitivity to these antigens.[48] More significantly, dogs immunized with gastric juice not only developed autoantibodies but also cell-mediated immunity to gastric antigens.[49] These animals had positive cutaneous delayed hypersensitivity and inhibition of leukocyte migration within 2 weeks of immunization. At that stage, there was evidence of atrophic gastritis; autoantibodies appeared a few weeks later, suggesting that cellular hypersensitivity may have caused the mucosal damage, with antibodies appearing as a secondary phenomenon. Nevertheless, the precise role of cell-mediated immunity in pernicious anemia remains speculative, and much further work is required.

B. Type B Atrophic Gastritis

Type B atrophic gastritis is more common than type A, though less is known about its pathogenesis. It is distinguished from type A by involving the antral mucosa. Its incidence increases with age, and it is more common in the lower socioeconomic groups; patients with type B gastritis are often symptomatic, and the lesion may predispose to peptic ulcer disease.

Vandelli et al.[50] have described antibodies to the gastrin-secreting antral G cells in a small percentage of patients whose sera were also negative for gastric parietal cell canalicular and intrinsic factor antibodies. In this respect, it may be pertinent that the G cell mass was reduced in these patients.

Rosen et al.[51] examined the possibility that type B gastritis was an allergic disorder by showing that many such patients had significantly elevated serum IgE levels. Furthermore, one quarter of the gastritis patients had specific IgE antibodies to food allergens. IgE plasma cells were also increased in the gastric lamina propria, the highest levels tending to be found in those patients with specific food antibodies. This latter observation suggests that, at least in a subgroup of these patients, food allergy may play an important role. Whether this response is due to mucosal damage with increased permeability to dietary antigens or whether it is a primary event has yet to be determined.

Of great interest is the recent description of spiral bacilli in the stomachs of patients with chronic gastritis.[52,53] Though first recognized as spirochetal organisms in 1906, their role has remained in doubt. Doenges[54] considered the organisms to have a pathogenic role in gastric disease. With the advent of gastroscopy and improved microbiological methods, their possible significance is now being explored. Though these organisms are found in a small number of healthy people, and in patients with various other gastric diseases, they are isolated most commonly in patients with gastritis. They occur on the surface of the gastric mucosa, in the necks and bases of gastric glands, and also beneath the mucous layer, where presumably they are protected from acid.

The organisms have been identified as Campylobacters (provisionally *Campylobacter pyloridis*) and are particularly found in antral gastritis. At the site of identification the mucosa shows acute as well as chronic inflammatory changes, suggesting that they are not merely commensals. One exciting possibility is that these organisms have antigens shared with gastric epithelium, predisposing them to mucosal damage. As yet there have been no studies on this aspect or indeed on whether these organisms elicit an immune response.

C. Varioliform Gastritis

This condition, also known as verrucous gastritis and chronic erosive gastritis, was only described as recently as 1976 by Andre and co-workers,[55] and though it was initially thought to be very rare, it is being recognized increasingly. It is an inflammatory condition which affects the fundus, body, and particularly the antrum of the stomach. It is easily identified at endoscopy when small erythematous nodules with shallow central erosions (''octopus sucker gastritis'') are found in association with swollen gastric rugae.[56] The radiological appearances are also characteristic, showing many nodules 3 to 11 mm in diameter, each with a central collection of barium situated along the rugal folds.[57]

Patients present with epigastric pain, anorexia, weight loss, nausea, and vomiting and rarely gastrointestinal bleeding; in most, the disease is chronic, with remissions and exacerbations, though about 17% recover spontaneously.[56]

The condition can occur after treatment with nonsteroidal, anti-inflammatory drugs. In some patients, symptoms improve with antacids.

On histology, there is superficial mucosal ulceration, an inflammatory infiltrate in the lamina propria consisting predominantly of plasma cells, and enlargement of the glandular structures with preservation of specialized cells.

Varioliform gastritis is considered to have an allergic basis mainly involving type I immediate hypersensitivity for a number of reasons. It has a typical relapsing clinical course; the atopic disorders, eczema, asthma, and urticaria are common,[58] and many patients have peripheral blood eosinophilia. Serum IgE can also be elevated,[59] but of most significance is the finding of large numbers of IgE plasma cells in the gastric lamina propria.[58,60] Though there is an overall increase in plasma cells, including IgA-staining cells, the increase in IgE plasma cells is most striking (40 to 60 times that of controls). Cell kinetic studies suggest that excessive histamine release causes the characteristic gastric gland hyperplasia.[60]

On treatment with sodium cromoglycate, patients show clinical, endoscopic, and histological improvement with a reduction in the number of IgE plasma cells in the lamina propria.[59,60] As sodium cromoglycate blocks the release of the inflammatory mediator histamine, 5-HT, and SRS-A from activated mast cells, this is further evidence of an allergic basis to this disease. Furthermore, sodium cromoglycate is significantly more effective than H_2 receptor antagonists in healing the gastric erosions.

To date, no specific allergen has been identified as an etiological agent in varioliform gastritis. In an animal model using *Mastomys natalensis* (a mast cell-rich African rodent), gastric intramucosal injection of ovalbumin in presensitized animals causes mucosal anaphylaxis.[61] A similar process involving dietary antigens could occur in humans. In summary, it is thought that patients with varioliform gastritis have an excess of IgE plasma cells in their gastric mucosa and are hypesensitive to one or more food allergens. On exposure to the allergen(s), specific IgE induces disruption of mast cells with release of histamine, which then stimulates acid release. In addition, histamine causes altered mucosal resistance and direct tissue injury. One consequence of this is an increase in macromolecule absorption with further tissue damage. A vicious cycle ensues, culminating in erosive gastritis. Identification of specific allergens will be required before this hypothesis can be verified.

D. Eosinophilic Gastroenteritis

Eosinophilic gastroenteritis is characterized by gastrointestinal symptoms and signs, peripheral blood eosinophilia, and eosinophilic infiltration of the gastrointestinal tract following the ingestion of specific foodstuffs. Though it is usually considered to be due to food allergy, other specific allergens such as penicillins may also cause the syndrome.[62]

The stomach and small intestine are the usual organs affected with patchy involvement, but eosinophilic infiltration has also been described in the esophagus, colon, pancreas, bladder, and gall bladder.[63] Histology shows marked eosinophilic infiltration of the lamina propria in those patients with mucosal disease. Uncommonly, the muscularis or serosa may be affected.[64]

Symptoms consist of postprandial nausea and vomiting, abdominal pain, weight loss, and diarrhea. When the muscularis is involved, intestinal obstruction can occur and also, very rarely, ascites from serosal involvement. Ankle edema is not uncommon due to hypoalbuminemia from a protein-losing enteropathy. Charcot-leyden crystals are found in the stools, and with small intestinal involvement, malabsorption also occurs with mild steatorrhea and occasionally impaired xylose absorption. Iron-deficiency anemia due to gastrointestinal blood loss is common. Patients have a peripheral blood eosinophilia which may be up to 50% of the total white cell count. Endoscopy shows hyperemic, edematous gastric folds, most marked in the pylorus, while radiology is nonspecific showing just prominent rugae.

Serum IgE levels are elevated in some patients.[65] Occasionally, IgE antibodies to specific foods are detected by RAST, and these correlate with positive skin tests to the particular food. In the majority of patients, however, the specific allergens remain unidentified. Other tests of immune function, such as levels of Ig and complement and total lymphocyte counts are normal.[63] T cell function as assessed by the response to phytohemagglutinin (PHA), concanavalin A (Con A) and pokeweed mitogen (PWM) is also normal. Elimination diets are helpful both in identifying the allergen and in treating the condition, but on the whole, correlation between the response to elimination diets and the results of specific skin tests is poor. In patients who do not respond to such a diet, an elemental diet may be more successful. Most patients will, however, respond to steroids, and in this respect, ACTH may be more beneficial than prednisolone.[62] The role of disodium cromoglycate remains to be established.

On the basis of recent studies the pathogenesis of this condition may now be postulated. IgE antibody to specific dietary or other antigens in the presence of this antigen binds to mast cells and basophils. This results in the release of preformed mediators such as leukotrienes and 5-hydroxyeicosatetraenoic acid (5HETE) and a eosinophil chemotactic factor of anaphylaxis (ECF-A). Leukotriene-B4 and 5-HETE attract eosinophils to the site of their reaction (chemokinesis), while ECF-A with histamine cause them to remain at the site. These substances also increase the expression of C3B receptors on the eosinophil. Eosinophils possess eosinophil cationic protein, eosinophil major basic protein, and eosinophil protein X which are toxic to cells;[66] for example, these proteins can kill schistosomules of *Schistosoma mansonii*.[67] Eosinophils have IgE receptors that take part in cytotoxic reactions.[68] After stimulation with complexed C3-6 or IgG, the eosinophils degranulate.[69]

The combination of cytotoxic factors released from eosinophils and the humoral mediators of inflammation released by mast cells and basophils result in the tissue damage and symptoms seen in eosinophilic gastroenteritis.

III. CELIAC DISEASE

The exact mechanism whereby gluten damages the jejunal musoca in celiac disease is still unknown. Initially it was considered to be due to a peptidase deficiency, which by allowing toxic metabolites of gliadin to accumulate resulted in intestinal damage.[70] No such enzyme deficiency has been discovered; however, considerable evidence of immunity to gluten has accumulated since the Frazer et al. historic studies.[70]

As already described in Chapter 1 a characteristic of untreated celiac disease is the increased number of intraepithelial lymphocytes in the jejunal mucosa,[71] a high proportion of which are T cells.[72-75] After dietary gluten withdrawal their numbers fall,[73] and conversely, in patients with celiac disease on a gluten-free diet, intraepithelial lymphocytes increase after oral gluten challenge.[74] Also, in the lamina propria of celiacs on a normal diet, lymphocytes are decreased and plasma cells increased. On gluten withdrawal, the number of lymphocytes increase toward normal, and there is a concomitant fall in plasma cells.[73]

Also suggestive of immunological mechanisms being of importance is the effect of steroids in celiac disease. It has long been known that steroids will ameliorate the adverse effects of gluten[76-78] and can induce a clinical remission.[79] In an in vitro organ-culture system, Falchuk and Katz[80] have also shown that cortisol reduces the total amount of Ig secreted by celiac jejunal mucosa. In addition, Katz et al.[81] have demonstrated that jejunal mucosa from untreated celiac patients remains abnormal if cultured in the presence of gluten but reverts toward normal when cultured with gluten and cortisol.

Other features indirectly suggesting abnormal immunity in celiac disease are the finding of splenic atrophy, atrophy of peripheral nodes but hypertrophy of mesenteric nodes, and the increased incidence of malignancy.[82]

A. Humoral Immunity

Patients with untreated celiac disease have elevated serum levels of IgA[83] and reduced levels of IgM.[84] These return toward normal on gluten withdrawal. In the lamina propria, there is an increase in plasma cells producing all classes of Ig, though the most marked increase is in IgA and IgM plasma cells.[85] Increased levels of IgA, IgM, and IgG are also found in the intestinal juice,[86] while IgA is found in the serum of celiac patients significantly more often than in patients with inflammatory bowel disease, and higher values are found in those on a normal diet compared with patients on a gluten-free diet.[87] Nonetheless, IgA, either local or systemic, is not essential in the causation of celiac disease, as celiac disease is well described in patients with selective IgA deficiency.[82] In fact this deficiency is approximately ten times more common in patients with celiac disease than in the general population.

Concerning antibodies, serum antibodies to wheat protein and gluten are present in patients with celiac disease.[88,89] However, these antibodies are not disease specific; also, celiacs have antibodies to a number of other foods besides wheat, and their presence probably reflects nonspecific macromolecular absorption due to increased intestinal permeability. Likewise, antibodies to gluten fraction III have been found in the upper intestinal secretions of celiac patients[90] but again are not disease specific.[89]

Antibodies to crude gliadin are invariably found in children with untreated celiac disease.[91,92] These predominantly IgG class antibodies are also found in 50% of children with other gastrointestinal diseases; IgA antigliadin antibodies have also been described in children with celiac disease.[93]

More convincing data are provided from studies using purified gliadin fractions; α-gliadin, a purified wheat protein, is more toxic to celiac jejunal mucosa, both in vivo and in vitro than crude wheat preparations or other gliadin fractions.[94,95] In this respect, O'Farrelly and co-workers[96] detected antibodies to α-gliadin by an enzyme-linked immunosorbent assay and found significantly higher titers in patients with untreated celiac disease than in healthy controls or in patients with inflammatory bowel disease. On a strict gluten-free diet, antibody titers fell into the normal range. The humoral response to α-gliadin may therefore have pathogenic significance, as well as a role as a diagnostic test.[97] Of related interest is the fact that celiac peripheral blood mononuclear cells show significant binding with a monoclonal antibody to α-gliadin compared with controls.[98,99] Further studies looking at patients with other gastrointestinal diseases are needed before the specificity of this reaction can be ascertained.

Circulating antigen-antibody complexes have also been detected in 40% of untreated celiac patients using a CIq assay[100] but in only 2% using RAJI cells.[101] Using Ciq-binding assays, Bullen et al.[102] Hall et al.,[103] and Corazza et al.[104] found circulating immune complexes in 12.8, 18.2, and 16.7% of celiacs, respectively. The composition of these complexes is unknown, and in any case there is no evidence that they are of pathological significance. In fact such complexes may represent a physiological way of clearing food protein antigens.[105]

IgG-class antireticulin antibody was first described in 36% of the patients with celiac disease in 1971.[106] However, it was subsequently found to occur in Crohn's disease and less commonly in other intestinal diseases.[107,108] IgA-class antireticulin antibody does appear to be more specific;[109] IgA antibodies are found in 79% of celiacs and 13% of controls.[110] The IgA antireticulin antibody is also found in jejunal secretions of untreated celiac patients, rarely in those of treated patients, and not in healthy controls,[111] so presumably it is produced locally in the gastrointestinal tract of celiac patients. The role of the reticulin antibody in celiac disease is unknown; the antibody is actually directed against a number of components of connective tissues, namely, endothelial basement membrane, perivascular connective tissue, epithelial basement membrane, and glomerulus.[112]

Local humoral immune mechanisms are undoubtedly involved in the immune response to gluten. When celiac patients in remission are challenged with gluten, there is increased synthesis of IgM and IgA by the jejunal mucosa.[113] A large proportion of this IgM and IgA represents antigluten antibody,[114] though IgG is also involved.[115] Furthermore, after gluten challenge, complement-fixing IgA complexes are found along the basement membrane of jejunal mucosa.[116] It is likely that after exposure to gluten, these antigen-antibody complexes damage the enterocyte. This may be dependent on the presence of a particular HLA haplotype on the cell surface.

Finally, type I, immediate hypersensitivity was initially considered unimportant in the pathogenesis of celiac disease, however, some recent studies suggest it may play some part. There is an increase in jejunal mucosal mast cells (MMC) in untreated celiac disease, which reverts to normal on a gluten-free diet. Furthermore, following gluten challenge, early mast cell degranulation occurs in the jejunum.[117] Using a modifed immunoperoxidase technique, they also found highly significant increases in IgE plasma cells in untreated celiac jejunal mucosa, falling to normal on treatment. Furthermore, McLaughlin and co-workers[118] demonstrated that, following challenge with α-gliadin in vitro, jejunal mucosa from patients with celiac disease released histamine. On this basis it has been suggested that reaginic hypersensitivity to gluten causes "leakiness" of the jejunal mucosa, allowing subsequent type II, III, and IV immune reactions. Further studies are necessary to confirm and expand these findings. It is of interest, in this respect, that the incidence of asthma and skin atopy are significantly increased in patients with celiac disease.[119]

B. Cell-Mediated Immunity

Over the past decade there has also been great interest in the role of cellular hypersensitivity in the pathogenesis of celiac disease. The condition can occur in the presence of profound antibody deficiency, thus Webster et al.[120] have described a patient with common variable immunodeficiency who had celiac disease and responded to a gluten-free diet. Further confirmation that this was celiac disease came from the studies of Marsh and Haeney,[121] who found a raised mitotic index in the patient's jejunal mucosa, which they considered to be specific to celiac disease. Antibody-mediated mechanisms are not therefore necessarily the prime cause of mucosal damage. Studies of cell-mediated immunity have concentrated on the response of peripheral blood lymphocytes to various fractions of gluten, direct studies of the jejunal mucosa, and skin testing.

1. Lymphocyte Studies

The leukocyte migration inhibition test has been most widely used as an indicator of delayed hypersensitivity to gluten in patients with celiac disease. Douwes[122] first demonstrated leukocyte migration inhibition to gluten in a group of 12 celiac patients but not in patients with a variety of other gastrointestinal diseases. Using α-gliadin, Haeney and Asquith[123] found that leukocyte migration inhibition occurred in 80% of celiacs on a gluten-free diet, 37.5% of celiacs on a normal diet, and only 3.7% of nonceliacs. Antigen specificity was also shown. The lower response rate in celiacs on a normal diet (i.e., containing gluten) may have been because activated T cells home preferentially to the gut in these patients and therefore are not detected in peripheral blood. Bullen and Losowsky,[124] using gluten fraction III, produced similar results. This test is even more specific in children; Ashkenazi and colleagues[125] found that 94% of celiac children produced leukocyte migration inhibition in the presence of a gluten subfraction.

A percentage of their children became negative to the test on a prolonged gluten-free diet, suggesting either a reduction in the number of sensitized cells or possibly the development of specific suppressor cell activity.

Using a modification of this test with direct assay of lymphokine production, O'Farrelly et al.[126] found that all 8 untreated celiacs and 14 of 15 treated celiacs produced lymphokine in the presence of α-gliadin (compared with only 2 of 28 controls). Simpson and co-workers[127] also confirmed that leukocyte migration inhibition to gluten occurs in celiac patients; however, they additionally found a similar degree of inhibition in HLA-B8 positive nonceliac controls. In this respect, it has been suggested that there is an immune response gene for gluten in linkage disequilibrium with HLA-B8, and as more than 80% of celiacs possess this antigen, a positive test could indicate the presence of this antigen. Furthermore, Simpson et al.[128] presented evidence that the gluten-induced leukocyte migration inhibition test in celiac disease may be measuring the effects of cytophilic antibody rather than lymphokine production. This latter work needs confirmation, and further studies are required on the exact mechanisms of leukocyte migration inhibition in celiac disease.

Lymphocyte transformation has been used to detect cellular hypersensitivity to specific antigens but with variable results in celiac disease. Ansaldi et al.[129] and Morganroth et al.[130] were unable to demonstrate blast transformation in the peripheral blood lymphocytes of patients with celiac disease when cultured with gluten. However, Holmes et al.[131] using higher concentrations of gluten fraction III, found evidence of cellular hypersensitivity in 29% of celiacs on a normal diet and 52% of those on a gluten-free diet.

C. Jejunal Mucosa

Many of the observations suggesting cellular hypersensitivity in celiac jejunal mucosa are derived from morphological studies including the finding of increased numbers of intraepithelial lymphocytes already alluded to.[132] In a number of detailed studies, Marsh[133-135] has also shown that in jejunal mucosa from patients with untreated celiac disease, these lymphocytes are blast transformed and highly mitotic. It has been alleged that this raised mitotic index is specific to celiac disease, and Marsh and Haeney[136] have also postulated that these immunoblasts are sensitized to gluten and provide further evidence of a local cell-mediated reaction to gluten. The pretreatment jejunal mucosal appearance of villous atrophy and crypt hyperplasia has also been cited as evidence of a local type IV reaction because rats infected with *Nippostrongylus brasiliensis* develop similar features,[137] and in other T lymphocyte induced-intestinal illnesses, namely, graft vs. host disease or allograft rejection, comparable mucosal changes are also found.[138,139] There are, however, important differences between these animal studies and the findings in untreated celiac disease. In particular, the enterocytes are preserved in the animal models, whereas they are characteristically abnormal in untreated celiacs.

Finally, the most direct evidence of local cell-mediated immunity to gluten in celiac disease was provided by Ferguson and co-workers.[140] In this study, celiac jejunal mucosa cultured in vitro in the presence of α-gliadin produced the lymphokine, macrophage migration inhibition factor, indicating the presence of a population of lymphocytes sensitized to α-gliadin in the mucosa. However, as with the peripheral blood studies, the exact type of cell producing the lymphokine has not yet been identified.

D. Skin Testing

Intradermal skin testing to detect delayed hypersensitivity to gluten has largely been unsuccessful in celiac disease. Thus Asquith,[141] using gluten fraction III, found no macroscopic abnormality in 20 of 21 celiacs at 48 hr. Baker and Read,[142] also using gluten fraction III, had positive reactions in 52% of untreated celiacs and 33% of gluten-free celiacs. However, these reactions were deemed Arthus type and not examples of delayed hypersensitivity. Likewise, Rawcliffe et al.[143] found positive arthus reactions with gluten subfraction B2 in all celiacs studies and sadly in a high percentage of patients with inflammatory bowel disease and controls. There are a number of possible explanations for not finding delayed hypersensitivity reactions in the experiments described; for example, the correct antigenic fraction of gluten may not have been used.

E. Genetic Studies

There is an increased familial incidence of celiac disease, with 5 to 20% of relatives being affected.[144] The role of the HLA system has been extensively studied in celiac disease both with regard to the genetic aspects and to explain gluten toxicity. The well-known association between HLA-A1 and B8 haplotype was described in the early 1970s, these antigens being found in only 20 to 25% of the normal population but in 75% or more of celiac patients.[145,146] Subsequently, an even higher association was described for HLA-DR3, 80% of celiacs compared to 20 to 30% of healthy controls.[147] HLA-A1 and B8 are associated through high linkage disequilibrium with DR3. The allele HLA-DR7 is also increased,[148] and in fact, if a patient possesses both DR3 and DR7, there is an even greater risk of having celiac disease. This association of celiac disease with two DR loci is rather unusual in that most other diseases are associated with only a single DR allele.

It was evident that HLA antigens alone could not account for the susceptibility to celiac disease, as 20% of the population possess the HLA-B8 or DR3 antigens and are not celiacs. In this respect, the description of a "gluten-sensitive enteropathy (GSE) B cell antigen" by Mann et al.[149] is very interesting. This B lymphocyte marker is found in 75 to 80% of celiacs but only in 6 to 18% of healthy controls; it was also found in 100% of parents of celiac patients. Celiac disease occurred when a person was homozygous for this B cell antigen and in addition possessed HLA-DR3 or an antigen in association with DR3. The GSE-associated B cell antigen is distinct and separately inherited from the HLA antigens;[150] that is, there are at least two genes controlling celiac disease. It was suggested that these two genes act cooperatively, possibly coding for proteins which make up a single structure on the surface of the lymphoid cells. Supporting this hypothesis are the animal studies of Kagnoff.[151] In this mouse model, two separate genetic regions determine the antibody response to α-gliadin, namely, the H2 region on chromosome 17 (the murine equivalent of the HLA region) and the Ig heavy chain allotype locus on chromosome 12. The H2-linked genes were the main determinants of the antibody response to gliadin. Variable region-idiotypic determinants on the Ig heavy chain cooperate in this response, either by cellular cooperation, or by their involvement in lymphocyte receptor recognition of specific antigens such as gliadin.

Of even greater interest is the recent description by Tosi et al.[152] that celiac disease is associated with a DC locus allele. Within the structure of the HLA-D region, two loci known as SB and DC also control allo-antigenic specificities. These are closely linked to the DR locus, and one specific allele, DC3, is in strong linkage disequilibrium with DR 3 and DR7. In their study of 60 patients with celiac disease, 59 possessed either HLA-DR3, DR7, or DR3 + DR7. All 60 patients possessed the DC allele. It was therefore suggested that DC3 is the HLA specificity primarily associated with celiac disease and that the association with DR3 and DR7 is because of their linkage disequilibrium with DC3. In a further study of children with gluten intolerance, Elliott et al.[153] found the DC3 allele in all the children who were proven to have celiac disease.

F. Immune Pathogenesis of Celiac Disease

The precise means by which hypersensitivity to gluten causes celiac disease and also why only a tiny proportion of the millions of people who eat gluten develop celiac disease is still not fully known. Nevertheless, over the last 20 years, interest has been focused on celiac disease as an immune disease. On the basis of the data already presented, a number of immunopathogenetic mechanisms have been proposed.

There is considerable evidence that a local humoral immune response occurring in the jejunal mucosa plays an important role. In tissue culture experiments, jejunal mucosa from patients with untreated celiac disease is further damaged by exposure to gluten, whereas that from patients with treated celiac disease is not. Furthermore, if jejunal mucosa from treated celiacs is cocultured in vitro with jejunal mucosa from untreated celiacs, then on exposure to gluten, the "remission" celiac mucosa becomes susceptible to the toxic effects of gluten.[154] This suggests that (1) gluten activates an effector mechanism to induce mucosal toxicity and (2) that the jejunal mucosa of patients with untreated celiac disease produces humoral factors or sensitized cells which can mediate tissue damage. Gluten does bind to jejunal mucosal epithelial cells in celiac patients.[155-157] In addition, immunocytes which produce antibody and which bind gliadin are also found in the lamina propria of celiac jejunal mucosa.[158]

Numerous studies have shown that patients with celiac disease have serum antibodies to gluten and its subfractions. Antibodies to α-gliadin bind to epithelial cells,[99,115] and following exposure to gluten, there is complement consumption and deposition of immune complexes in the subepithelial tissues producing tissue damage.[159,160]

There is also much evidence that cell-mediated immunity is important in effecting mucosal damage. The intraepithelial lymphocytes, so prominent in untreated celiac disease are mainly T lymphocytes of the cytotoxic/suppressor variety.[132] Furthermore, a significant proportion of these lymphocytes are blast transformed and highly mitotic, and on a gluten-free diet, these changes revert to normal.[133,136] This suggests that these lymphocytes are responding to a luminal antigen, namely, gluten. In fact, on exposure to gluten in vitro, untreated jejunal mucosa produces the lymphokine, the macrophage migration inhibition factor. This is further evidence of local cellular hypersensitivity to gluten (though the actual cells producing the lymphokine are not yet known). The production of this lymphokine by peripheral blood lymphocytes after exposure to gluten and various subfractions thereof has been confirmed on a number of occasions.

The humoral and cellular mechanisms described above probably work in cooperation, and in this regard, it is presently thought that the HLA system plays a central role. Both HLA-B8 and DR3 are associated with generalized immune hyperresponsiveness and are found in a number of autoimmune diseases. Furthermore, healthy HLA-B8 controls show more marked in vitro lymphocyte transformation to wheat antigens than B8-negative subjects.[161] Likewise nonceliac B8-positive individuals show a similar degree of leukocyte migration inhibition to gluten, as do celiac patients.[127] It seems likely therefore that a specific immune response gene linked to HLA-B8 and/or DR3 facilitates the specific immune response to gluten seen in the jejunal mucosa in celiac disease. Alternatively, the histocompatibility genes may code for the production of cell surface proteins which function as receptors. As the majority of people with HLA-B8 and/or DR3 do not develop celiac disease, other factors must be implicated. The non-HLA-linked, GSE B cell antigen may be involved here. Falchuk[162] has proposed that patients with celiac disease have cell surface proteins coded for by both histocompatibility antigen genes and the B cell antigen. The occurrence of HLA-B8/DR3 and the B cell antigen would lead to the formation of a receptor for gluten on the enterocyte or intestinal lymphocyte. Following binding of gluten to the epithelial cell surface receptor, it becomes a target for local mucosal immune responses, either the production of antigluten antibodies, lymphokines, or both. The resulting cytotoxicity would lead to epithelial cell damage and the consequent features of celiac disease.

The very strong association of HLA-DC3 with B8, DR3, and DR7 and with celiac disease offers a further approach to pathogenesis. The DC locus may control induction of T cell-specific killing. (This has already been shown for DC1.) In this event, HLA-B8 and DR3 would be recognized because of their linkage disequilibrium with DC3, though DC3 would be of prime importance, most likely by initiating cellular cytotoxicity. Nonetheless, other loci must also be involved, as 30% of the general population possess this antigen. The likely candidates are the GSE B cell antigen or an Ig heavy chain marker. More work is clearly necessary to confirm and extend these findings.

Finally, an attractive alternative hypothesis regarding the causation of celiac disease is that gluten is acting as a toxic lectin.[163] Lectins are naturally occurring proteins and glycoproteins which can agglutinate erythrocytes and certain other cells because of their ability to bind, sometimes with high specificity, carbohydrate residues on the cell surface. Interaction of a plant lectin with exposed reactive sites (such as an incomplete glycoprotein) can cause changes leading to cell toxicity and death. Weisar and Douglas[163] suggested that in celiac disease there is an abnormal increase in incomplete glycoproteins on the small intestinal cell surface membrane. Douglas[156] had previously described a gluten fraction (glyc-gli) which could bind to a crude membrane fraction of celiac intestinal mucosa but not to a similar fraction of normal mucosa. Thus in celiac disease, gluten or one of its subfractions could bind to alter exposed, incomplete cell surface membrane glycoproteins and act as a toxic lectin, which would alter cell function, resulting in earlier death and therefore increased cell turnover. The emerging cells would be less differentiated and less mature and therefore have more cell surface membrane-incomplete glycoproteins with a further increase in gluten binding sites, resulting in eventual total villous atrophy. The basic metabolic defect in this hypothesis is an increase in incomplete oligosaccharide chains not normally associated with the surface membrane glycoproteins of the mature epithelial cells. The subsequent clinical and immunological features of celiac disease are quite compatible with this basic pathogenetic model.

Experimental support for the lectin hypothesis was provided by the animal studies of Lorenson and Olsen.[164] They demonstrated that a wheat germ lectin can cause enterocyte damage with resultant villous atrophy and crypt hypertrophy. This was related to the ability of the lectin to bind to carbohydrate residues. Kottgen and co-workers[165] confirmed that gluten has lectin-like properties and that glycoproteins from immature small intestinal crypt cells are more reactive than those from the mature villous zone. They suggested that in celiac disease, increased gluten binding could be due to the presence of a high proportion of oligomannosyl-glycoproteins in the brush border membrane and that this is due to a genetically determined deficiency of the growth-dependent *N*-acetyl-glucosaminyl transferase-I. Further work is presently in progress utilizing these models, and the results could alter our perception of the pathogenesis of celiac disease, and offer some novel approaches to treatment.

IV. CMPI

CMPI is essentially a disease of childhood and includes a number of syndromes which result from intolerance to one or more cow's milk proteins. One of the most important is cow's milk protein enteropathy, in which the sensitivity causes reversible small intestinal abnormalities and malabsorption.[166] There is evidence for an immunological basis to these syndromes. Hypolactasia with lactose intolerance is also very common in childhood. It may result from a number of insults to the gastrointestinal tract, e.g., infection, or be hereditary. It will not be discussed further, though it may occur in association with CMPI. The incidence of CMPI is not accurately known, partly because of its protean manifestations and partly because of differing diagnostic criteria. Goldman and co-workers[167] suggested a figure of 12% Frier and Kletter[168] suggested 0.5%, and Gerrard and co-workers[169] suggested 7.5%. The most recent estimates indicate that CMPI affects 1 to 3% of children.[170]

A. Clinical Features

Symptoms which follow milk ingestion can be gastrointestinal or less commonly systemic and be immediate or delayed. The resulting illness may be acute or chronic.

CMPI affects infants, usually within the first 6 months of life, and symptoms usually disappear by 1 to 2 years. In the acute syndrome, vomiting after cow's milk ingestion is the usual manifestation. Infants with cow's milk protein enteropathy have malabsorption with diarrhea, vomiting, weight loss, and failure to thrive.[166] The milk intolerance is a transient finding unlike the lifelong sensitivity found in celiac disease. Infantile colitis may also be due to CMPI: Jenkins and colleagues[171] described eight children less than 2 years old with bloody diarrhea and an acute "colitis" on rectal biopsy. These children had a family history of atopy, and all had eosinophilia and elevated serum IgE levels. The symptoms appeared shortly after the first introduction of cow's milk and improved on its elimination. In those who were rechallenged with cow's milk, the colitis recurred. These authors claimed that food allergy, in particular to milk, was the cause of most if not all colitis in children less than 1 year old. This is a particularly interesting finding in the light of the suggestion by Whorwell et al.[172] that ulcerative colitis (but not Crohn's disease) in adults is associated with a history of childhood bottle feeding.

The diagnosis of cow's milk protein enteropathy is confirmed by intestinal biopsy and diagnostic milk challenge.[173] Biopsy at presentation shows either partial or subtotal villous atrophy.[166] The child is then placed on a milk-free diet, and a further biopsy is performed when the infant is clinically improved, at which stage the jejunal mucosa should be normal. The child is then given milk "under supervision" and the biopsy repeated. In those with enteropathy, the mucosa will once again become abnormal, thus confirming the diagnosis. These children often become symptomatic following the challenge, with diarrhea, vomiting, weight loss, and occult gastrointestinal bleeding. This procedure is definitive and supersedes older techniques such as the Goldman criteria.[167] It also excludes other diseases such as giardiasis and celiac disease, which may mimic cow's milk protein enteropathy.

Generalized symptoms in CMPI include urticaria, wheezing, and eczema; anaphylaxis is fortunately rare.[174] However, Parrish and colleagues[175] have suggested that cot death may be due to anaphylaxis to cow's milk. It was postulated that the infant becomes sensitized to cow's milk following oral administration. Should such a child regurgitate and then aspirate milk during sleep, anaphylactic bronchoconstriction with death could follow. Certainly, this can occur experimentally in guinea pigs.[176] If this were the explanation in humans, there should be evidence of a latent anaphylactic sensitivity in otherwise healthy infants. McLaughlin and Coombs[177] have indeed found that 25% of infants have this as assessed by basophil histamine release following milk challenge. On this basis, the use of hypoallergenic milk formulas could result in less sensitization, and this would be of profound practical significance.

Babies can also be sensitized to substances eaten by mothers and excreted in breast milk. Gerrard and Shenassa[178] described 73 breast-fed babies who developed a number of symptoms such as colic, vomiting, diarrhea, rhinorrhea, bronchitis, eczema, and urticaria. In 61 children, this was due to sensitivity to cow's milk ingested by the mother and excreted in breast milk. Symptoms were relieved by the mother avoiding cow's milk. These babies had positive skin sensitivity and IgE RAST tests to cow's milk protein and were presumably sensitized to trace amounts of the antigen.

B. Immunology of CMPI

Virtually all infants fed cow's milk develop milk antibodies, though in the majority there are no clinical consequences.[179] IgG antibodies appear first, reaching a maximum at 3 to 4 months, while IgA antibodies appear more slowly, not peaking until 7 months. IgM antibodies are found in only minimal quantities.[180] Infants with CMPI have significantly fewer IgA-staining plasma cells in the lamina propria than healthy infants or children with celiac disease; this may well be relevant to the pathogenesis of the condition.[181,182] Intestinal SIgA is in any event low in neonates and infants, and milk precipitins and immune complexes containing milk protein are found in over half of patients with selective IgA deficiency.[183] It is this combination of mucosal and systemic IgA deficiency that is probably of prime importance in "predisposing" to mucosal injury in CMPI.

The subsequent immunopathogenesis of CMPI is still not fully understood, but there is evidence of type I, III, and IV reactions in different circumstances.

1. Type I

The clinical course in many infants with CMPI is suggestive of an immediate hypersensitivity, type I, reaction. Reactions occur soon after ingesting milk, and in addition to diarrhea and vomiting, these infants may also develop urticaria, angio-edema, eczema, rhinitis, and anaphylaxis. Dannaeus and Johnsson[184] found 71% of patients showing immediate reactions had positive skin tests and specific IgE RAST antibodies to milk.[184] Similarly, Ford and colleagues,[185] who used strict Goldman criteria to confirm CMPI (i.e., three blind milk challenges each eliciting characteristic symptoms), found a proportion of their patients had immediate reactions often to small quantities of milk. These patients had cutaneous manifestations, positive skin tests, raised serum IgE, and specific IgE antibodies to milk. Furthermore, after a milk challenge, the number of mucosal IgE-producing plasma cells increase.[181,186] In an important description by Pearson,[184] it was shown that in 11 of 16 children with CMPI some plasma cells produce specific antibody to β-lactoglobulin or bovine serum albumin; 70% of these cells were IgA, and 30% were IgE class. This is therefore direct evidence of local production of IgE to milk protein in these patients. Whether this locally produced IgE can fix to mast cells and mediate intestinal damage remains to be proven. The local reaction could increase intestinal permeability, allowing further antigen entry and access to the systemic circulation and hence eliciting a systemic immune response. This latter could account for the distant effects such as urticaria, bronchospasm, etc.

2. Type III

Type III, immune complex-mediated, hypersensitivity may be implicated in relatively delayed reactions to cow's milk protein.[185] These infants have negative skin tests and no specific IgE milk antibodies and require larger quantities of milk to provoke symptoms. Circulating immune complexes can be detected in most infants after feeding milk.[188] Thus Frick[189] and Paganelli and co-workers[190] showed that after a milk challenge, controls, atopic patients, and milk allergic subjects had immune complexes containing β-lactoglobulin. However, these were of IgA class in the nonatopic patients and probably of protective value. In contrast in the milk allergic subjects, IgE and IgG complexes were also found; these patients also had CIq-binding complexes. It was suggested that in milk-allergic subjects, mixed IgG and IgE complexes bind CIq and activate the classical pathway, resulting in clinical symptoms.

Elevated titers of IgG and IgA milk antibodies have been found in milk sensitivity.[191]

In antigen excess, these could elicit a type III response. The presence of an associated type I reaction with IgE antibodies would favor the local deposition of these immune complexes.

3. Type IV

Delayed hypersensitivity, type IV, reactions are likely to be of importance in those children with CMPI whose symptoms occur 24 to 48 hr after ingestion of cow's milk. These children show lymphocyte blast transformation in the presence of milk antigen[192,193] and evidence of lymphokine production.[194] The jejunal villous atrophy in CMPI has also been cited as evidence of a delayed reaction.[195]

In summary type I, III, and IV responses are all likely to be of importance in CMPI, the particular component differing in different children. Jackson et al.[182] suggested one model for the pathogenesis of CMPI based on the fact that many of these illnesses follow an acute gastrointestinal infection. By damaging the small intestinal mucosa, this causes increased permeability to dietary antigens such as milk. Because of functional immaturity, the small intestine cannot adequately respond, and in addition, many of these infants have a transient IgA deficiency, which further predisposes them to excess antigen entry. Indeed, utilizing horseradish peroxidase uptake studies, increased amounts of unprocessed antigen have been shown to enter the damaged small intestinal mucosa. A type I reaction occurring at the mucosal surface with the ensuing capillary dilatation would further increase intestinal permeability, with entry of antigen to the systemic circulation. Subsequent local and systemic immune responses (types I, III, and IV) would determine the type and site of the pathological process and be manifested as clinical illness. On a milk-free diet the systemic immune response would gradually abate, and with increasing maturity of the local immune system, the vulnerability to intestinal infection and mucosal permeability would diminish, hence the transient nature of CMPI. It is of interest in this respect that infants with CMPI possess similar HLA antigens to the general population.[196]

V. SOYA PROTEIN ENTEROPATHY

Soya protein is ubiquitous in the Western diet. It is a nutritious and generally safe food; in fact its initial popularity stemmed from its supposed "hypoallergenic" properties. However, there have been a number of reports of generalized and gastrointestinal allergic reactions in both children and adults.

Soya protein enteropathy was first described by Ament and Rubin[197] in 1972 in a child who developed diarrhea, vomiting, dehydration, and a metabolic acidosis after exposure to soya protein. On three subsequent occasions following oral soya protein challenge, jejunal biopsies showed subtotal villous atrophy. There was an initial neutrophil infiltration of the lamina propria succeeded by a lymphocyte and plasma cell infiltrate at 24 hr features which improved within 96 hr. Following the challenges, precipitins to soya protein were detected in serum. Soy bean isolate was shown to be the cause of villous atrophy, with no response occurring to gluten, cow's milk or soy bean lecithin. A very similar case was described by Goel et al.[198] in 1978.

In 1977, Whittington and Gibson[199] described four children with concomitant soya and CMPI. The dual sensitivities were confirmed by Goldman's criteria, though biopsies were not performed. It was postulated that the cow's milk sensitivity first damaged the gut mucosal barrier, allowing subsequent absorption of soya allergens with resulting soya hypersensitivity. In the more detailed clinical description of Kuitenen and colleagues,[166] 54 patients with CMPI were recorded. Of these infants, 35 received soya protein as a milk substitute, of whom 4 developed concomitant soya protein hypersensitivity. Jejunal biopsy showed partial villous atrophy in three and subtotal villous atrophy in the fourth. Morphometric studies in five additional children with combined CMPI and soya protein intolerance showed that the jejunal mucosal response to soya protein was identical to that seen in celiac disease after gluten challenge.[200]

During soya challenge, the number of IgA and IgM plasma cells increased, whereas IgG and IgE plasma cells were unchanged. Sufficiently long-term follow-up studies have not been performed in children with soya protein enteropathy to state whether it is a transient or permanent disorder.

A. Pathogenesis of Soya Protein Enteropathy

In animals, pathogenesis of soya protein enteropathy has been clearly defined by Barrett et al.[201] Serum hemagglutinating antibodies to soya protein were detected in calves within 7 days of commencing a soya-based diet. The levels were extremely high and more typical of hyperimmunization than of a casual response to dietary antigen. The younger the calf, the higher the antibody response, suggesting that to some extent immaturity of the gastrointestinal tract was implicated, with low levels of SIg synthesis and impaired antigen exclusion. However, even in older calves, the local gut immune mechanism was only partially successful in excluding antigen absorption, as significant levels of soya protein antibody were also found in this group. The predominant antibody was of IgG1 subclass, which could precipitate with soya protein extracts and activate complement, so eliciting a type III hypersensitivity response. Morphological changes in the small bowel of the animals similar to the human cases also occurred, with villous atrophy and increased mononuclear cell infiltrate in the villi and lamina propria. However, other immunological findings in humans have been nonspecific, and whether the mechanism in man is a type III hypersensitivity remains to be proven.

The initiating factor in soya protein hypersensitivity in infants displaying this alleged type III response could be defective chemotaxis. Butler and co-workers[202] found that infants with soya protein intolerance had a significant decrease in chemotaxis compared with healthy controls and conversely had significantly increased random migration of neutrophils. An immature permeable mucosal barrier in these infants could allow intact proteins to gain access to the circulation, followed by a local and systemic immune response. Previous animal studies on the role of neutrophils in these circumstances[203] had demonstrated the movement of neutrophils in large numbers to the small intestine of weaning pigs which had been immunized and then enterally exposed to the immunizing antigen. If an antigen penetrated the epithelial surface of the gut, the resulting emigration of neutrophils to the site would eliminate that antigen. However, in the presence of an impaired neutrophil response, e.g., depressed chemotaxis (as described in soya-sensitive children),[202] the antigen could gain access to the circulation and elicit an immune response.

B. Soya Protein Hypersensitivity in Celiac Disease

Up to 10% of celiac patients show a suboptimal response to a gluten-free diet.[204] This condition has been termed "nonresponsive celiac disease," or refractory sprue,[205] and a number of factors have been suggested to account for this poor response. These include failure to maintain dietary gluten exclusion, impaired mucosal DNA synthesis, subepithelial collagen deposition,[206] associated zinc deficiency,[207] and coexistent hypersensitivity to other foods.

As the Barrett et al. studies[201] have shown, soya protein can induce intestinal mucosal damage in animals by immunologically mediated hypersensitivity. Patients with celiac disease are particularly exposed to soya, as the protein is commonly used as a gluten substitute in gluten-free diets. Studies from Birmingham have suggested that a coexistent hypersensitivity to soya protein is a significant cause of the suboptimal response to gluten withdrawal seen in some celiac patients. Of 84 adult patients with celiac disease, 12 were identified who showed a poor response to gluten withdrawal.[208]

These patients remained symptomatic and had persisting hematological and biochemical abnormalities and malabsorption after 2 or more years on a strict gluten-free diet. Morphometric analysis of their jejunal biopsies, while showing some improvement on a gluten-free diet, nonetheless showed significantly less improvement than that seen in celiacs who had shown a good clinical response to gluten withdrawal. Furthermore, significant levels of antisoya protein antibodies were detected in the celiac group when compared with healthy controls and patients with duodenitis and inflammatory bowel disease, with the highest titers in the poorly responsive celiacs.[209] This was unlikely to be simply due to increased mucosal permeability from persisting jejunal villous damage, as there was no correlation between antisoya antibodies and antibodies to other common dietary antigens in these poorly responsive celiacs.

In a further study, cell-mediated immunity to soya protein was also assessed in these patients utilizing the leukocyte migration inhibition test.[210] Significantly lower migration indexes to soya were found in the poorly responsive celiacs than in celiacs who were on a normal diet (i.e., untreated), in those who had shown a good response to a gluten-free diet, or in control groups of healthy subjects, patients with inflammatory bowel disease, or with a variety of other upper gastrointestinal diseases.

Having demonstrated humoral and cellular immunity to soya protein in these poorly responsive celiacs, 10 of the 12 patients were placed on a diet excluding soya protein as well as gluten. Reassessment after 6 months showed clinical improvement, a return to normal of hematological and biochemical parameters and normal intestinal absorptive capacity.[208] Of particular interest were the biopsy findings; jejunal morphometry showed significant improvement and was indistinguishable from that seen in celiacs who had shown a good response to a gluten-free diet alone. Concomitant with this histological improvement, there was a diminution in the immune response to soya protein.

Thus a significant number of patients with celiac disease who show a poor response to gluten withdrawal have a coexistent immunological hypersensitivity to soya protein which may compromise their response to the gluten-free diet. Soya protein could also induce or perpetuate intestinal mucosal damage in celiac disease by acting as a toxic lectin in the way suggested for gluten by Weisar and Douglas.[163] The subsequent immune response would then further damage the intestinal mucosa.

VI. INFLAMMATORY BOWEL DISEASE

The pathogenesis of inflammatory bowel disease, i.e., Crohn's disease and ulcerative colitis, remains unknown. A number of pathogenetic mechanisms have been suggested including autoimmunity, toxic environmental factors, genetic susceptibility, infection, and diet. Recently, however, immunological processes have been studied in most detail. Overall, there is a marked increase in immunological reactivity in inflammatory bowel disease, particularly directed against the gastrointestinal tract. Whether this activity causes the disease or whether it is a secondary phenomenon perpetuating the inflammatory process has yet to be resolved. Though the immunological findings in Crohn's disease and ulcerative colitis are broadly similar, they will be considered individually.

a. Crohn's Disease

1. Immunological Etiology

There is an undoubted familial predisposition to Crohn's disease with an increased risk of 30-fold in siblings and 13-fold in other first degree relatives.[211] This could indicate a genetically determined abnormal immune hyperresponsiveness.

There have been reports of Crohn's disease in association with autoimmune diseases, e.g., pernicious anaemia.[212] Nonetheless, there has been no overall increase in tissue autoantibodies in populations with Crohn's disease, and the associations with autoimmune disease are therefore probably chance occurrences.[213,214] Four patients with Crohn's disease and arthritis have also been found to have anti-idiotypic antibodies, which in other contexts are thought to have a role in autoimmune disease.[215] Much more information is, however, required on this antibody before its significance in Crohn's disease can be determined. Similarly, in a study by Stocker and colleagues,[216] 36% of patients with Crohn's disease had autoantibodies to pancreatic acini, compared with only 5% of ulcerative colitis patients and 3% of controls. The nature and significance of this antibody is also unknown. The extraintestinal manifestations of Crohn's disease such as iritis, arthritis, and erythema nodosum are similar to those found in serum sickness, suggesting an immune-complex-mediated illness. In fact immune complexes have been detected in such patients but are more likely to be secondary to the intestinal lesion.[217]

Immune competence in Crohn's disease has been generally found to be normal; hypogammaglobulemia,[218] and selective IgA deficiency[219] are, in practice, rare occurrences. Serum Igs are usually normal or raised,[219] and there is a rise in circulating SIgA.[220] Increased synthesis and turnover of Igs[221] and of the C3 component of complement[222] have been noted, while numbers of peripheral blood lymphocytes are reduced,[223] normal,[224] or increased.[225] More recent work by Sieber and co-workers[226] has found markedly raised numbers (tenfold) of spontaneous Ig secreting cells in patients with active Crohn's disease, indicating a high degree of polyclonal B cell activation.

In Crohn's disease, an overall impairment of cell-mediated immunity has long been recognized, including a degree of cutaneous anergy, though individual reports have differed. Thus a high percentage of patients with Crohn's disease do not respond to intradermal tuberculin,[227] though other studies have denied this.[228] DNCB, a potent skin sensitizer in healthy people, elicits a response in only 50% of patients with Crohn's disease. Impaired cellular reactivity to other antigens has also been found in Crohn's disease.[229,230]

Similarly, in vitro tests of T lymphocyte function have given conflicting results. Reduced responsiveness has been found to PHA and Con A.[230-233] However, normal responses to PHA have also been recorded.[141,233] These differences are partly explained by differences in technique and partly by the choice of controls. If ill, as opposed to healthy, controls are used, then the differences are no longer significant.[233] Zinc deficiency, commonly found in Crohn's disease, has also been considered to contribute to the impaired cellular immunity, but in fact mononuclear cell levels of zinc are normal.[234] Malnutrition can also impair delayed hypersensitivity and is obviously a very important modulator in different studies; monocyte suppressor cells may also be relevant. Kelleher et al.[235] showed that with pure lymphocyte cultures from patients with Crohn's disease there was enhanced transformation; however, it was reduced in mononuclear cell cultures (as used in previous studies). There is a relative monocyte excess in active Crohn's disease, and monocytes can suppress lymphocyte transformation by prostaglandin production, suggesting that a monocyte suppressor cell may partly determine this response.

Numbers of circulating T lymphocytes and other lymphocyte subpopulations have been assessed using conventional and monoclonal markers. The absolute number of T cells have been reported as normal[233] or decreased,[225,236] while T cell subsets show normal values.[237] Godin and co-workers[238] found normal ratios of T_h to T_s cells in patients with inactive Crohn's disease or those on steroids. During disease activity, however, there was a reversal of the T_h to T_s cell ratio due to a decrease in suppressor/cytotoxic cells. Serial studies also showed these alterations in the T_h to T_s cell ratios to coincide with episodes of disease activity. These observations could be explained if suppressor/cytotoxic T cells are pooled at the site of injury in the gut wall during disease exacerbations. There is also some variability in reports of T cell function. Both spontaneous and Con A-induced T_s cell activity in peripheral blood has been described as reduced.[219,239] Yet other studies have found either normal[226,240] or even increased T_s activity.[241]

Nevertheless, T_h cell function appears normal. These findings in peripheral blood may or may not reflect what is happening at the mucosal level, which is of prime importance. Whether they are of pathogenic significance also remains to be determined.

2. The Mucosal Lesion

In Crohn's disease, the lesion is one of transmural inflammation with increased numbers of immunocompetent cells, namely, plasma cells and lymphocytes. Noncaseating granulomata are also found in 60% of patients. Macroscopically, the bowel is affected in a segmental, discontinuous fashion, with intervening apparently normal areas of gut. However, on microscopy, even these "normal" areas show inflammatory changes (see also Chapter 1 [Volume I]).

In normal intestinal mucosa, IgA class, B lymphocytes and plasma cells predominate with only moderate numbers of IgG- and IgM-producing cells. In contrast, in the inflamed mucosa from patients with Crohn's disease, there is an increase in all Ig-containing cells. The increase in IgG plasma cells is most marked relative to moderate increases in IgM cells, and there are only slight increases in IgA cells.[242-244]

Excess IgM-producing cells are found throughout the gastrointestinal tract in Crohn's disease,[245] the increase occurrring irrespective of disease activity; it is not found in ulcerative colitis.[246] The IgM cells are close to the surface epithelium, whereas the excess IgG cells are found deeper in the lamina propria.[244] These changes are probably due to different functional roles of these cells in Crohn's disease. Intestinal B lymphocytes produce Ig; Bookman and Bull[247] found a tenfold increase in IgG synthesis but normal IgA synthesis. Conversely, MacDermott et al.[248] found reduced spontaneous production of IgG, IgA, and IgM in vitro compared with controls, IgA production being the most affected. Verspaget and co-workers[249] recorded results similar to Bookman and Bull and also found spontaneous Ig production from peripheral blood and lamina propria lymphocytes to be greater in Crohn's disease than in controls. Additionally, in Crohn's disease, Ig synthesis was greater in intestinal lymphocytes compared to peripheral blood lymphocytes, and PWM reduced Ig production from lamina propria lymphocytes, while increasing it in peripheral blood lymphocytes. Overall this suggests that the lamina propria lymphocytes in Crohn's disease are a unique activated cell population. The role of the locally synthesized antibodies is as yet unknown, though they could be directed against dietary antigens, intestinal organisms, or even cell surface antigens. In particular, immune complexes have not been found in the intestinal mucosa to date, though there are data to make one suspect that they are involved in the pathogenesis of Crohn's disease.

T lymphocytes are increased in Crohn's disease mucosa mainly in the lamina propria.[250] This discounts intraepithelial lymphocytes, the majority of which are cytotoxic/suppressor cells and whose individual numbers are unaltered.[251] The ratio of T_h cells to T_s cells as assessed by monoclonal antibodies (OKT4 and OKT8) is normal in Crohn's disease,[234,251] whereas in vitro results of T_s cell activity have given discrepant results. Normal suppressor function was found by Shorter[252] and Fiocchi and colleagues,[253] but reduced suppressor function was found by Goodacre and Bienenstock.[254] On the other hand, Fiocchi et al.[255] in a more detailed study have found enhanced T_s cell activity in inflammatory bowel disease (both Crohn's disease and ulcerative colitis). Some of these discrepancies are due to lack of standardization of the control groups and hence firm conclusions cannot be drawn.

Intestinal mononuclear cells from Crohn's disease patients proliferate in the mixed lymphocyte reaction to the same degree as healthy controls.[248] These cells therefore possess receptors which can recognize foreign cell surface antigens. Likewise, Crohn's disease lymphocytes demonstrate normal cytotoxic reactions in vitro.[256]

Killer (K) cells which are involved in antibody-dependent cellular cytoxicity (ADCC) and natural killer (NK) cells which do not require antibody can be detected by the monoclonal antibody LEU-7. Using this technique, K and NK cells are uncommon among intestinal mononuclear cells, approximately 0.3 to 3.0%.[257] They are found in the lamina propria and also lymph follicles. Furthermore, K cell activity has been found in mononuclear cells from mesenteric lymph nodes (MLN) in patients with active Crohn's disease but not from normal controls.[258]

3. Macrophages and Neutrophils

Macrophages are found in the inflammatory infiltrate in Crohn's disease, especially in active disease.[247] They are particularly found in the granulomata, the hallmark of Crohn's disease, suggesting that these cells have an important role in the pathogenesis of this condition. Kinetic studies of macrophage turnover in Crohn's patients indicate that this is a low-turnover granulomatous state (comparable to sarcoidosis).[259] Interestingly, the rate of turnover is similar in both Crohn's disease and ulcerative colitis. The monocytes show normal bacterial killing in Crohn's disease, while phagocytosis is increased compared with healthy and disease controls.[260,261]

Macrophage migration in Crohn's disease is normal, as demonstrated by the skin-window technique.[262] The intestinal macrophages also show normal motility and a normal response to chemotactic stimuli.[263] The random motility of monocytes has been found to be increased, while monocyte chemotaxis is similar to controls in Crohn's disease, though increased in ulcerative colitis.[264]

Blood monocytes from Crohn's subjects are activated with increased lysosomal enzymes,[265] the increase correlating with disease activity. Serum activity of the lysosomal enzymes is also increased but is not related to disease status. The intestinal macrophages also show an increase in lysosomal enzyme activity, which may be important in the disease process.[266] In Crohn's disease the monocytes release increased quantities of plasminogen activator, a neutral proteinase which generates plasmin with resulting tissue damage.[267] Also, Ligumsky and co-workers[268] have demonstrated the production of prostaglandins E2 and I2 and thromboxane A2 by inflamed rectal mucosa, presumably reflecting the increased numbers of monocytes present.

In 1977, Ward[269] suggested that a defect in macrophage function in Crohn's disease impairs the handling of particulate and antigenic material, leading to granuloma formation. However, the above studies demonstrate that the monocytes are more active in Crohn's disease, and there is no intrinsic functional defect. This increased activity, both in serum and in the intestine, presumably reflects activation by the underlying disease process. How these monocytes are stimulated and their exact role in the inflammatory process remain to be determined. Nonetheless, their function is altered by drugs commonly used in Crohn's disease, e.g., sulfasalazine[270] and corticosteroids.[271]

In contradistinction to the macrophages, the polymorph leukocytes show reduced migration into the skin window.[272] There are other signs of neutrophil dysfunction, such as an impaired nitroblue tetrazolium reaction during phagocytosis[273] and impaired luminescence.[274] Verspaget and co-workers[275] have also demonstrated defective production of hydrogen peroxide in neutrophils of patients with untreated Crohn's disease, whereas this was normal in treated Crohn's disease, indicating a partial intrinsic cellular defect impairing the production of oxygen metabolites. Whether this is a primary process or a secondary effect remains to be determined. In combination with the abnormalities of neutrophil motility, this metabolic dysfunction could lead to impaired clearances of foreign material and might therefore contribute to granuloma formation.

4. Humoral Responses

Circulating autoantibodies to colonic epithelial cells appear in Crohn's disease, though less frequently than in ulcerative colitis.[276,277] These antibodies cross-react with colonic and certain *Escherichia coli* antigens. To date, however, these antibodies have not been directly shown to cause damage to the colonic epithelium, and there is no correlation between their titers and the extent or activity of disease, raising doubts about their significance. Though there is a great increase in mast cells in the inflamed mucosa in Crohn's disease, there is no evidence of a type I hypersensitivity to colonic mucosa.[278]

Levels of antibody to dietary antigens such as milk protein and gluten are similar to controls,[279] though antibodies to bovine serum albumin are increased;[280] specific IgE antibodies to foods are also raised.[281] Whether these dietary antibodies are of pathogenic significance is debatable, since only a small proportion of patients with inflammatory bowel disease respond to treatment with sodium cromoglycate.

Circulating immune complexes have also been found in the sera of patients with Crohn's disease,[282,283] especially if the disease is in remission or associated with complications such as arthritis. Using a conglutinin-binding ELISA (enzyme-linked immunosorbent assay), McKenzie and co-workers[284] have shown that both IgG and IgA complexes occur and are heterogenous in size. Complement is found in the tissues in Crohn's disease,[285] and there is evidence of complement consumption.[283] Despite all these features suggesting a type III hypersensitivity reaction, precipitated immune complexes have not been described in the intestinal mucosa.

5. Cell-Mediated Immunity

Those histological features of small intestinal Crohn's disease manifested by increased intraepithelial lymphocytes and crypt length in the jejunum at the site of focal fissures, ulcers, or granulomata are consistent with a local cell-mediated reaction.[286] In this respect, Fiocchi and co-workers[287] have shown that isolated T cells from the mucosa in active Crohn's disease form 60% stable E-rosettes in tissue culture compared to less than 10% in controls or inactive Crohn's patients, also suggesting activated T cells in Crohn's disease.

Dykes[288] demonstrated leukocyte migration inhibition to small intestinal contents in Crohn's disease. Inhibition could also be obtained using homogenated diseased colonic epithelium, the degree of inhibition varying with disease activity[289] in contrast to the earlier work of Bendixen,[290] who also used colonic epithelium but with negative results. Using the different technique of lymphocyte transformation, however, cellular hypersensitivity to colonic cells[291] or intestinal contents[292] could not be demonstrated. Patients with Crohn's disease, nevertheless, do show cell-mediated immunity to the common enterobacterial antigen of Kunin.[293] Also Crohn's disease intestinal mononuclear cells show enhanced proliferation to lipopolysaccharide (LPS) and *Staphylococcus aureus* antigens, but not to other bacterial antigens, suggesting that activated T lymphocytes are present in the intestinal mucosa.[287]

Finally, Crohn's peripheral blood lymphocytes are cytotoxic to colonic epithelial cells but not to ileal cells.[294] Serum factors are involved, and the effector cell has neither T nor B cell characteristics, raising the possibility that this is an example of

ADCC.[295] In this respect it is to be recalled that Britton and co-workers[258] have demonstrated the presence of ADCC in mesenteric node mononuclear cells from patients with active Crohn's disease.

6. Other Factors in the Pathogenesis of Crohn's Disease

a. Infection

As stated earlier there is an undoubted familial predisposition to Crohn's disease which could indicate a genetically determined hyperresponsiveness. It is not, however, associated with any specific histocompatibility antigen.[296-298] An infective agent might therefore underly the pathogenesis of Crohn's disease: however, epidemiological studies do not support this view. Thus in large well-controlled studies, no space-time clustering has been found[299] nor has there been any increase in "effective contact" between patients when compared with controls.[300] Also, there is no increase in Crohn's disease in medical staff who are in constant contact with Crohn's patients. Furthermore, antibodies to anerobic coccoid rods, which are commonly found in patients with inflammatory bowel disease, are not found in attending medical staff.[301]

Nonetheless, because of the presence of granulomata in Crohn's disease, many studies have looked for mycobacterial infection; no such organism has been found.[302] Similarly, searches for *Yersinia*[303] and *Chlamydia*[304] have been negative. Because Crohn's tissue homogenated can induce cytopathic effects in tissue culture cells, a viral etiology has been considered. Gitnick and co-workers[305] showed that these cytopathic effects could be serially passed on in sensitive culture lines and apparently identified a responsible virus. This work, however, could not be reproduced by Yoshimura and co-workers,[306] who demonstrated that this transmissible factor was not a virus but was in fact a nonreplicating cytotoxic factor which could be released from intestinal tissues of patients with and without inflammatory bowel disease. Despite all these negative or contradictory findings, much work continues in trying to identify an infectious agent in Crohn's disease.

b. Diet

The role of diet in the pathogenesis of Crohn's disease has also received much attention. The finding of food antibodies in such patients has already been mentioned. Regarding specific foodstuffs, James[307] suggested that Crohn's disease may be associated with eating cornflakes. However, these findings could not be confirmed by others.[308,309] An increased consumption of refined carbohydrates has also been noted in Crohn's patients[310] but not in ulcerative colitics.[311,312] Heaton and co-workers[313] have in fact treated patients with Crohn's disease with a diet containing unrefined carbohydrate but rich in fiber, with subsequent improvement in the patients' condition. Whether this improvement is simply due to the diet-altering gut flora is unknown.

Other specific food intolerances have been identified by Hunter et al.[314] in a number of Crohn's patients. The most common foods implicated were wheat, dairy products, and corn. In a subsequent controlled trial, 29 of 33 patients with active Crohn's disease were identified as having specific food intolerance.[315] Avoidance of specific foods led to prolonged remission in 21 of these 29 patients, with improvement in the disease activity index. In terms of food allergy, Tschaikowski[316] found a high incidence of sensitization to mold allergens which contaminate food. Using a combination of desensitization and elimination diet, an apparent permanent remission was achieved in 36 of 49 patients with Crohn's disease. The findings from both of these studies if confirmed by others could be of great importance concerning the pathogenesis and treatment of Crohn's disease.

c. Smoking

Following the reports that nonsmoking was associated with ulcerative colitis, Logan and colleagues[317] looked at the incidence of smoking in Crohn's disease. Before their disease onset, Crohn's patients were significantly more likely to be smokers than age- and sex-matched controls, and smokers carried an increased relative risk of developing Crohn's disease. The reason for this is unknown, but it is of interest that smoking is associated with an increased consumption of refined sugar and can also affect immune function.

B. Ulcerative Colitis

1. Immunological Etiology

Many of the findings relating to the immunology of ulcerative colitis are similar to those already described in Crohn's disease. There is a genetic predisposition to ulcerative colitis, with 10 to 29% of patients having an affected relative.[297,318] Analysis of numerous family studies does not suggest a Mendelian inheritance, and there is no association with HLA-A or B antigens.[319] However, the HLA-DR2 antigen appears to be increased in ulcerative colitis,[320] and there may also be a negative association with HLA-DR7. As with Crohn's disease there are isolated case reports of ulcerative colitis occurring in autoimmune diseases such as systemic lupus erythematosis[213] and pernicious anemia.[212] However, these are probably coincidental chance associations, and overall there is no significant increase in tissue autoantibodies in ulcerative colitis subjects.[321]

Extraintestinal manifestations, i.e., arthritis, iritis, and erythema nodosum, also occur in ulcerative colitis, suggesting an immune complex-mediated process. Indeed, it has been suggested that endotoxin entering the circulation from the inflamed colon activates complement at the site of the lesion.[322]

Other parameters relevant to the humoral immune system in ulcerative colitis are generally unaltered. Serum Ig are unremarkable,[219] whereas the complement components C3 and C4 and factor B are generally normal but increase in those with active disease.[217,323] Both synthesis and catabolism of C3 and Clq are also increased,[217,324] and C3 breakdown products are formed in active ulcerative colitis,[325] indicating complement activation, possibly by locally produced immune complexes.

Cell-mediated immunity is less affected in ulcerative colitis than in Crohn's disease. The ratio of T to B cells is not altered.[326] As in Crohn's disease, there is a decrease in absolute numbers and relative proportions of suppressor/cytotoxic (OKT8) cells during disease activity.[238] This fall is sufficient to cause a fall in the total T lymphocyte count. In fact, Strickland et al.[326] had previously noted a T lymphopenia during active disease. During remission or on steroid treatment, absolute numbers of T cells and the T_h to T_s cell ratios are normal, and it is likely that during disease exacerbations T_s cells are sequestered in the inflamed colon. Curiously and without obvious explanation, splenic atrophy is found in ulcerative colitis,[327] being more common in long-standing disease. In this regard, it therefore resembles celiac disease.

Tests of nonspecific cell-mediated immunity in ulcerative colitis have given variable results. Delayed hypersensitivity skin testing has been reported as normal.[328] Conversely, Ainley and co-workers.[234] found impaired cutaneous hypersensitivity to similar recall antigens. Furthermore, Binder et al.[328] showed normal cutaneous sensitization with DNCB, whereas Meyers et al.[329] found an anergic reaction. In vitro lymphocyte transformation with PHA has given a normal response in many studies.[292,330-332] However, Sachar et al.[231] obtained a depressed response in one third of their patients following PHA stimulation. Normal responses were obtained with Con A and PWM.[331] In contrast other workers found a reduced response to Con A, although at only suboptimal concentrations, and this was ascribed to an abnormal T_h to T_s cell ratio in ulcerative colitis.[234]

Overall, therefore, general immune function is preserved in ulcerative colitis. Though abnormalities occur, these are not as marked as in Crohn's disease and probably reflect activity of the disease rather than an innate defect of immune function.

2. The Mucosal Lesion

Ulcerative colitis is a mucosal disease, and it is uncommon for the inflammatory process to extend into the submucosa. There is an increase in lymphocytes, plasma cells, and polymorphs in the mucosa. Additionally, crypt abscesses, goblet cell depletion, and glandular distortion or branching are found. As in Crohn's disease, there is a great increase in plasma cells producing Ig,[243] the most marked being in IgG cells. In contrast to Crohn's disease, IgM cells are not so predominant, and this feature may help to distinguish the two.[246] Most studies have found normal numbers of IgE-containing cells[243,246,333] with the exception of Heatley and colleagues,[334] who found an increase. Concerning lymphocytes, the majority are T cells among which T_s cell numbers are normal[253] or increased.[255] As in Crohn's disease, normal numbers of NK cells are found.[257]

3. Macrophages

Many of the findings for macrophages in Crohn's disease are similar in ulcerative colitis. Although granulomata characteristically occur only in Crohn's disease, kinetic studies have shown a similar low-turnover macrophage state in both conditions.[259] Absolute monocyte counts are higher in ulcerative colitis than in Crohn's disease,[265] but phagocytic activity and bacterial killing are similar.[261] Directional chemotaxis of monocytes is increased in ulcerative colitis when compared with Crohn's disease and controls.[260,335] This may be accounted for by the presence of less mature, more mobile cells in ulcerative colitis due to higher monocyte turnover.[259]

Skin window techniques have shown normal accumulation of macrophages but decreased mobility of neutrophils.[336] Bookman and Bull[247] have demonstrated an increase in macrophages in the colonic mucosa in ulcerative colitis. Monocytes are also activated in ulcerative colitis with increased lysosomal enzyme activities, the latter correlating with activity of the colitis.[265] The overall findings for lysosomal enzymes and neutral proteases are similar in Crohn's disease and ulcerative colitis.

4. Humoral Responses

Circulating autoantibodies to colonic epithelial cells have been found in many patients with ulcerative colitis, especially children.[337] These are autoantibodies in that they can also be detected when using the patients own colon.[338] They are of IgG, IgM, or IgA class but not IgE.[278] In vitro studies have not shown this autoantibody to be cytotoxic to colonic epithelial cells.[339] There is no association between the presence of antibody and the degree of activity of the colitis.[276] These antibodies may in fact be cross-reactive with intestinal bacterial antigens; raised antibody titers to *E. coli* 014 are found in patients with ulcerative colitis,[340] and the colonic antibody can cross-react with the LPS of *E. coli* 014.[341] The antibodies may initially have had a protective role against bacteria and only subsequently cross-react with colonic mucosa, with resulting damage. Against this suggestion is the occasional finding of these antibodies in patients with noninflammatory colonic diseases.[342]

Locally produced antibody to bacteria within the colonic mucosa has also been demonstrated.[343] Reaction between such antigen and antibodies resulting in immune complexes could also initiate cellular damage. Certainly, circulating immune complexes are found in ulcerative colitis[282] which are of IgG or IgA class.[284] Whereas it is an attractive hypothesis to suggest that local deposition of immune complexes causes the inflammation in ulcerative colitis, such complexes have yet to be identified.

5. Cell-Mediated Immunity

In vitro studies have demonstrated cellular hypersensitivity to colonic epithelium in patients with ulcerative colitis, utilizing either the leukocyte migration inhibition test[290] or lymphocyte transformation.[344] In addition, these patients show cellular immunity to the common enterobacterial (Kunin) antigen[293,345] and to certain strains of *E. coli*.[346] Other evidence comes from the description by Selby et al.[251] of an increase in type 3 macrophages, expressing cell surface HLA-DR antigens.[251] These type 3 macrophages were not found in healthy colons, and it was suggested that they are activated in response to foreign antigen, with subsequent T cell macrophage interactions. The number of T_h and suppressor/cytotoxic T cells are also increased in active Crohn's disease. In this respect, Broberger and Perlmann[339] have shown that lymphocytes from patients with inflammatory bowel disease are cytotoxic to colonic epithelial cells grown in tissue culture. This cytotoxicity was found only in patients with inflammatory bowel disease, and was lost following colectomy.[252] This reaction involved humoral factors also, and the effector cells had the characteristics of NK-K cells, suggesting that this may be antibody-dependent cell-mediated cytotoxicity.[295] Though only found in patients with inflammatory bowel disease, it does not correlate with the degree of disease activity. Furthermore, it is found in patients with Crohn's disease whose lymphocytes are cytotoxic to colonic epithelial cells; cytotoxicity to ileal cells cannot be demonstrated,[252] raising serious doubts about the in vivo role of this mechanism.

6. Other Factors in the Pathogenesis of Ulcerative Colitis

a. Infection

To date, no specific organism has been found in ulcerative colitis. Enteropathogenic strains of *E. coli* are found more commonly in the stools of patients with ulcerative colitis, but these postdate the onset of symptoms and are unlikely to be the cause of the colitis.[347] However, *E. coli* isolated from such patients have invasive and adherent properties (on HELA cell monolayers) more often than those from controls. These properties may affect the pathogenicity of the *E. coli,* and in this respect Pinder and co-workers[348] have shown these organisms to attach to colonic epithelium in vitro, the most marked adhesion being seen in colonic biopsies from patients with active ulcerative colitis. This may still of course be a secondary phenomenon.

The role of viruses in ulcerative colitis also remains speculative. Cave and colleagues[349] reported successful animal transmission studies in ulcerative colitis. Furthermore, Gitnick et al.[350] have shown that tissue homogenates from ulcerative colitis patients have cytopathic effects on tissue culture cells. These cytopathic effects could be serially transmitted in animals, and virus-like particles could be identified in the affected tissue culture cells, suggesting a viral etiology. In fact, these authors identified a 60-nM RNA-containing virus associated with ulcerative colitis. These results, however, could not be confirmed by others.[306,351] These three studies did find a cytopathic effect in tissue culture, but this was not specific, being also found in patients with other gastrointestinal diseases; it was not transmissible. Searches for cytomegalovirus[352] and adenovirus[353] have also been negative in ulcerative colitis.

In summary, based on these and numerous other studies, there is no evidence that a specific organism causes ulcerative colitis. Nonetheless, gut microorganisms appear to play a role in this condition, as evidenced by the development of humoral and cellular immunity directed against them. Whether the latter is a primary process or is secondary to inflammation is unknown.

b. Diet

The role of diet has been less well studied in ulcerative colitis than in Crohn's disease, with the exception of milk sensitivity. Wright and Truelove[354] showed that a percentage of patients with ulcerative colitis improved on milk-free diets and relapsed on exposure to milk. Hemagglutinating antibodies to milk are also found more frequently in such patients than in controls.[355] However, Jewell and Truelove[356] were unable to find specific IgE antibodies to milk and also found no increase in positive intradermal skin tests. Some patients with ulcerative colitis have hypolactasia with lactose intolerance which could also explain their improvement on milk exclusion. Food antibodies other than milk have been found in ulcerative colitis; Brignola and colleagues[357] found a higher incidence of specific IgE food antibodies to ten different foods in ulcerative colitis (12%) than in Crohn's disease (8%), or controls (1%). It remains, however, doubtful if these are of pathogenetic significance, and they may merely represent increased dietary absorption of the antigen secondary to mucosal damage.

c. Smoking

In 1982, Harries et al.[358] reported that patients with ulcerative colitis were less likely to smoke cigarettes than healthy controls. This has since been confirmed on a number of occasions;[359] only 18% of patients with ulcerative colitis are current smokers, compared with 32 to 38% of the population as a whole and 65% of patients with Crohn's disease. The excess of nonsmokers with ulcerative colitis is not due to life-long abstinence but to these patients having stopped smoking prior to developing their colitis.[360] The role of smoking in inflammatory bowel disease remains unknown. However, it has been suggested that these patients have a genetic predisposition to developing inflammatory bowel disease and whether they smoke or not will determine which type of disease they develop, i.e., Crohn's or ulcerative colitis, respectively.[317]

C. The Pathogenesis of Inflammatory Bowel Disease

The cause of inflammatory bowel disease is not known. Immunological mechanisms are probably of great importance in the associated tissue damage, but whether they are the prime instigator of this or are merely nonspecific effectors has yet to be determined.

The initiating agent may be infective (viral or bacterial), or some other toxic factor, perhaps a dietary antigen. This results in a damaged intestinal mucosal barrier, and consequently there is an increased absorption of dietary and infective antigens. At the mucosal level there is evidence of disordered immune regulation, and there may be abnormalities of effector cells. In any event, there is an increased humoral and cell-mediated immune response. This is directed against dietary, bacterial, viral, and other toxic gut associated antigens and is persistent. It involves specific immunocompetent cells with evidence for type I to IV hypersensitivity reactions and also nonspecific inflammatory mediators such as macrophages, neutrophils, and complement. Local alterations of immunoregulatory cells which modulate the immune response are probably of importance in perpetuating this process and in determining specific manifestations. The consequence of all this is a chronic inflammatory response with damage to the intestinal tract manifesting as Crohn's disease or ulcerative colitis. The extraintestinal manifestations are thought to be due to circulating immune complexes.

There are many gaps in this model of inflammatory bowel disease, and it does not explain the numerous different guises of the disease. There is a genetic susceptibility to this condition, which is not simple Mendelian inheritance or related to the histocompatibility antigens. Whether the patient smokes or not plays some part in the type of disease developed, though the mechanism for this is not known. Whether microorganisms are the cause of inflammatory bowel disease or whether they are absorbed because of the damaged mucosa and increased permeability and therefore play a secondary role has not been determined. This remains an area of active research, but results are often conflicting. The immune response is obviously of great importance in the tissue-damaging reactions but in the present state of knowledge is not enough to account for all the features of these two diseases.

VII. CONCLUSIONS

Based on these accounts, the evidence that immunological reactions are involved in certain human gastrointestinal conditions, namely, gastritis, celiac disease, CMPI, soya intolerance, Crohn's disease, and ulcerative colitis, appears overwhelming. However, it seems inconceivable that this would not be so, given the richness of the immunological apparatus of the human intestine reviewed elsewhere in this book; the gut associated lymphoid tissue was bound to be involved at some stage, whatever the nature of the initial insult. Although such immunological data have helped in our understanding of these diseases, of considerable disappointment is the continuing confusion regarding which of these immune reactions are primary and which are just epiphenomena. Also disappointing is our inability to answer the equally important question regarding the patient's own contribution to their hyperresponsiveness. It is admitted, however, that some progress has been made in this latter regard. The descriptions of disease in the rare immune deficiency states, e.g., the occurrence of gastritis in hypogammaglobulinemia, have helped our understanding of gastritis in those patients with normal humoral and cellular immune components. Celiac disease in IgA deficiency provides another example. Next is the information provided from genetic studies, e.g., of HLA antigens in celiac disease, with the further implication that these have regarding the patients immune hyperresponsiveness. This is obviously an area for further detailed study.

The nature of the external antigenic "insult" also requires greater definition but with at least one caveat. Even if we know the agent in all its molecular detail, this does not of necessity mean the disease will be fully understood. Thus we now know much more about which component of wheat is toxic in celiac disease, but our understanding of the mechanism of gluten toxicity has progressed independently of that biochemical detail. This then leaves clinicians and clinical immunologists with a sobering final thought. To the patient with celiac disease their main if not sole immediate concern is that gluten is toxic and that gluten withdrawal leads to normalization of health. They are unconcerned with the genetic basis for their hyperresponsiveness, the molecular composition of α-gliadin, the implications of the lectin hypothesis, etc. Should therefore more of our future efforts be directed to antigen identification but only in the broadest sense? Presumably, it is the greatest wish of the Crohn's patient or the sufferer from ulcerative colitis that we find the alleged infectious agent and destroy it.

REFERENCES

1. Strickland, R. G. and MacKay, I. R., A reappraisal of the nature and significance of chronic atrophic gastritis, *Am. J. Dig.*, 18, 426, 1973.
2. Lewin, K. J., Dowling, F., Wright, J. P., and Taylor, K. B., Gastric morphology and serum gastrin levels in pernicious anaemia, *Gut*, 17, 551, 1976.
3. Nerup, J., Cathelineau, C. R., Seignalet, J., and Thomsen, N., HLA and endocrine disease, in *HLA and Disease*, Dausset, J. and Svejgaard, A., Eds. Munksgaard, Copenhagen, 1977, 149.
4. Carmel, R. and Spencer, C. A., Clinical and subclinical thyroid disorders associated with pernicious anaemia, *Arch. Int. Med.*, 142, 1465, 1982.

5. Jewell, D. P. and Hodgson, H. J. F., Autoimmune and inflammatory diseases of the gastrointestinal tract, in *Immunological Aspects of the Liver and Gastrointestinal Tract*, Ferguson, A. and MacSween, R. N. M., Eds., MTP Press, Lancaster, 1976, 203.
6. Doniach, D., Roitt, I., and Taylor, K. B., Autoimmune phenomena in pernicious anaemia. Serological overlap with thyroiditis, thyrotoxicosis and systemic lupus erythematosis, *Br. Med. J.*, 1, 1374, 1963.
7. Feldt-Rasmussen, U., Bech, K., Bliddal, H., Hoier-Madsen, M., and Jorgensen, F., Autoantibodies immune complexes and HLA-D in thyrogastric autoimmunity, *Tissue Antigens*, 22, 342, 1983.
8. Wangel, A. G., Callender, S. T., Spray, G. H., and Wright, R., A family study of pernicious anaemia. I. Autoantibodies, achlorhydria, serum pepsinogen and vitamin B12, *Br. J. Haematol.*, 14, 161, 1968.
9. Mawhinney, H., Lawton, J. W. M., and White, A. G., HLA-A3 and HL-A7 in pernicious anaemia and autoimmune atrophic gastritis, *Clin. Exp. Immunol.*, 22, 47, 1975.
10. HLA and Disease Registry; Third report, Ryder, L. P., Andersen, E., and Svejgaard, A., Eds., Munksgaard, Copenhagen, 1979.
11. Carmel, R., Ozturk, G., Johnson, C. S., Tung, K. S., and Terasaki, P. L., Profiles of black and Latin American patients having pernicious anaemia, *Am. J. Clin. Pathol.*, 73, 291, 1981.
12. Van Den Berg-Loonen, E. M., Hilterman, C. H., Bins, M., Nijenhuis, L. E., and Engelfriet, P., Increased incidence of HLA-DR2 in patients with pernicious anaemia, *Tissue Antigens*, 19, 158, 1982.
13. Weissel, M., Hofer, R., Zasmeta, H., and Mayr, W. R., HLA-DR and Hashimoto's thyroiditis, *Tissue Antigens*, 16, 256, 1980.
14. Thomsen, M., Jorgensen, F., Brandsburg, M., Gimsing, P., Lanng-Nielson, J., Ryder, P., and Svejgaard, A., Association of pernicious anaemia and intrinsic factor antibody with HLA-D, *Tissue Antigens*, 17, 97, 1981.
15. Bardhan, K. D.,Wangel, A. G., Whitehead, R., Wright, R., Spray, G. H., Warner, G. T., and Callander, S. T. E., The relation between the histology of the gastric mucosa, secretion of intrinsic factor, autoimmunity and the absorption of vitamin B12, in *Protides of the Biological Fluids*, Proc. 16th Colloq. Bruges, Belgium, Preeters, H., Ed., Pergamon Press, Oxford, 1969, 393.
16. Samloff, I. M. and Turner, M. D., Rabbit blocking and binding antibodies to human intrinsic factor and intrinsic factor-B12 complex, *J. Immunol.*, 101, 57, 1968.
17. Samloff, I. M., Kleinman, M. S., Turner, M. D., Sobel, M. V., and Jeffries, G. H., Blocking and binding antibody to intrinsic factor and parietal cell antibody in pernicious anaemia, *Gastroenterology*, 55, 575, 1968.
18. Strickland, R. G., Baur, S., Ashworth, L. A., and Taylor, K. B., A correlative study of immunological phenomena in pernicious anaemia, *Clin. Exp. Immunol.*, 8, 25, 1971.
19. Goldberg, L. S. and Bluestone, R., Hidden gastric autoantibodies to intrinsic factor in pernicious anaemia, *J. Lab. Clin. Med.*, 75, 449, 1970.
20. Hoedemaker, P. J. and Ito, S., Ultrastructural localisation of gastric parietal cell antigen with peroxidase-coupled antibody, *Lab. Invest.*, 22, 184, 1970.
21. Masala, C., Smurra, G., Di Prima, M. A., Amendolez, R. A., Celestino, D., and Salsand, F., Gastric parietal cell antibodies: demonstration by immunofluorescence of their reactivity with the surface of gastric parietal cells, *Clin. Exp. Immunol.*, 41, 271, 1980.
22. De Aizpura, H. J., Toh, B. H., and Ungar, B., Parietal cell surface reactive autoantibody in pernicious anaemia demonstrated by indirect membrane immunofluorescence, *Clin. Exp. Immunol.*, 52, 314, 1983.
23. De Aizpura, H. J., Cosgrove, L. J., Ungar, B., and Toh, B. H., Autoantibodies cytotoxic to gastric parietal cells in serum of patients with pernicious anaemia, *N. Engl. J. Med.*, 309, 625, 1983.
24. Ward, H. A. and Nairn, R. C., Gastric parietal cell autoantigen; physical, chemical and biological properties, *Clin. Exp. Immunol.*, 10, 435, 1972.
25. Tai, C. and McGuigan, J. E., Immunologic studies in pernicious anaemia, *Blood*, 34, 63, 1969.
26. James, D., Asherson, G., Chananin, I., Coghill, N., Hamilton, S., Himsworth, R. L., and Webster, D., Cell mediated immunity to intrinsic factor in autoimmune disorders, *Br. Med. J.*, 4, 494, 1974.
27. Fixa, B. and Thiele, H. G., Delayed hypersensitivity to intrinsic factor in patients with pernicious anaemia, *Med. Exp. (Basel)*, 19, 231, 1969.
28. Fixa, B., Thiele, H. G., Komarkoua, O., and Nozicka, Z., Gastric autoantibodies and cell mediated immunity in pernicious anaemia: a comparative study, *Scand. J. Gastroenterol.*, 7, 237, 1972.
29. Weisbart, R. H., Bluestone, R., and Goldberg, L. S., Cellular immunity to intrinsic factor in pernicious anaemia, *J. Lab. Clin. Invest.*, 85, 87, 1975.
30. Finlayson, N. D. C., Fauconnet, M. H., and Krohn, K., In-vitro demonstration of delayed hypersensitivity to gastric antigens in pernicious anaemia, *Am. J. Dig. Dis.*, 17, 631, 1972.
31. Goldstone, A. H., Calder, G. A., Barnes, E. W., and Irvine, W. J., The effect of gastric antigens on the in-vitro migration of leucocytes from patients with atrophic gastritis and pernicious anaemia, *Clin. Exp. Immunol.*, 14, 501, 1973.

32. Kountouras, J., Raptopoulou-Gigi, M., and Goulis, G., A study of cell mediated immunity to gastric antigens in patients with atrophic type A and B gastritis, *Thymus*, 4, 173, 1982.
33. Whittingham, S., Youngchaiyud, U., MacKay, I. R., Buckley, J. D., and Morris, P. J., Thyrogastric autoimmune disease. Studies on the cell-mediated immune system and histo-compatibility antigens, *Clin. Exp. Immunol.*, 19, 289, 1975.
34. Katka, K., Immune functions in pernicious anaemia before and during treatment with vitamin B12, *Scand. J. Haematol.*, 32, 76, 1984.
35. Ungar, B., Whittingham, S., and Francis, C. M., Pernicious anaemia: incidence and significance of circulating antibodies to intrinsic factor and parietal cells, *Aust. Ann. Med.*, 16, 226, 1967.
36. Hughes, W. S., Brookes, F. P., and Conn, H. O., Serum gastrin levels in primary hypogammaglobulinaemia and pernicious anaemia, *Ann. Intern. Med.*, 77, 746, 1972.
37. Rose, M. S. and Chanarin, I., Dissociation of intrinsic factor from its antibody; application to study of pernicious anaemia gastric juice specimens, *Br. Med. J.*, 1, 468, 1969.
38. Rose, M. S. and Chanarin, I., Intrinsic factor antibody and absorption of vitamin B12 in pernicious anaemia, *Br. Med. J.*, 1, 25, 1971.
39. Inada, M. and Glass, G. B. J., Effect of prolonged administration of homologous and heterologous intrinsic factor antibodies on the parietal and peptic cell masses and the secretory function of rat gastric mucosa, *Gastroenterology*, 69, 396, 1975.
40. Hausamen, T. U., Halcrow, D. A., and Taylor, K. B., Biological effects of gastrointestinal antibodies. II. Histological changes in the stomach induced by injection of specific heterologous antibodies, *Gastroenterology*, 56, 1062, 1969.
41. Hausamen, T. U., Brus, I., Fisher, J. M., and Taylor, K. B., Inhibition of production of gastric acid by gastric antibodies, *Clin. Res.*, 17, 594, 1969.
42. Lovebridge, N., Bitensky, L., Clayen, J., Hausamen, T. U., Fisher, J. M., and Taylor, K. B., Inhibition of parietal cell function by human gammaglobulin containing gastric parietal cell antibodies, *Clin. Exp. Immunol.*, 41, 264, 1980.
43. Jacob, E. and Glass, G. B. J., The participation of complement in the parietal cell antigen-antibody reaction in pernicious anaemia and atrophic gastritis, *Clin. Exp. Immunol.*, 5, 141, 1969.
44. Te Velde, K., Hoedemaker, P. J., Anders, G. J. P. A., Arends, A., and Nieweg, H. O., A comparative morphological and functional study of gastritis with and without autoantibodies, *Gastroenterology*, 51, 138, 1966.
45. Tanaka, N. and Glass, G. B. J., Effect of prolonged administration of parietal cell antibodies from patients with atrophic gastritis and pernicious anaemia on the parietal cell mass and hydrochloric acid output in rats, *Gastroenterology*, 58, 482, 1970.
46. Kaye, M. D., Whorwell, J., and Wright, R., Gastric mucosal lymphocyte subpopulations in pernicious anaemia and in normal stomach, *Clin. Immunol. Immunopathol.*, 28(3), 431, 1983.
47. Jeffries, G. H., Recovery of gastric mucosal structure and function in pernicious anaemia during prednisolone therapy, *Gastroenterology*, 48, 371, 1965.
48. Andrada, J. A., Rose, N. F., and Andrada, E. C., Experimental autoimmune gastritis in the rhesus monkey, *Clin. Exp. Immunol.*, 4, 293, 1969.
49. Krohn, K. J. E. and Finlayson, N. D. C., Interrelations of humoral and cellular immune responses in experimental canine gastritis, *Clin. Exp. Immunol.*, 14, 237, 1973.
50. Vandelli, C., Bottazzo, G. F., and Doniach, D., Autoantibodies to gastrin-producing cells in antral (type B) chronic gastritis, *N. Engl. J. Med.*, 300, 1046, 1979.
51. Rosen, S. N., Bennett, M. K., Faux, J., and Jewell, D. P., Chronic gastritis — an allergic disorder? in *Proc. 2nd Fisons Food Allergy Workshop*, Medicine Publishing Foundation, Oxford, 1983, 73.
52. Marshall, B. J. and Warren, J. R., Unidentified curved bacilli in the stomach of patients with gastritis and peptic ulceration, *Lancet*, 1, 1311, 1984.
53. Rollason, T. P., Stone, J., and Rhodes, J. M., Spiral organisms in endoscopic biopsies of the human stomach, *J. Clin. Pathol.*, 37(1), 23, 1984.
54. Doenges, J. C., Spirochaetes in the gastric glands of *Macaca* rhesus and of man without related disease, *Arch. Pathol.*, 27, 469, 1939.
55. André, C., Moulinier, B., Lambert, R., and Bugnon, B., Gastritis varioliformis, allergy and disodium cromoglycate, *Lancet*, i, 964, 1976.
56. Lambert, R., André, C., and Moulinier, B., Diffuse varioliform gastritis, *Digestion*, 17, 159, 1978.
57. Elta, G. H., Fawaz, K., Dayal, Y., McLean, A., Phillips, E., Bloom, S. M., Paul, R. E., and Kaplan, M. M., Chronic erosive gastritis — a recently recognised disorder, *Dig. Dis. Sci.*, 28, 7, 1983.
58. André, C., Moulinier, B., André, F., and Daniere, S., Evidence for anaphylactic reactions in peptic ulcer and varioliform gastritis, *Ann. Allergy*, 51(2), 325, 1983.
59. André, C., Gillon, J., Moulinier, B., Martin, A., and Fargier, M. C., Randomised placebo-controlled double-blind trial of two dosages of sodium cromoglycate in treatment of varioliform gastritis: comparison with climetidine, *Gut*, 23, 348, 1982.

60. André, F., André, C., and Fournier, S., Measurement of glycoprotein content and cell kinetics in preulcerous gastric mucosa, *Dig. Dis. Sci.,* 24, 667, 1979.
61. André, F. and André, C., Gastric ulcer induced by mucosal anaphylaxis in ovalbumin sensitized praomys (mastomys) natalensis, *Am. J. Pathol.,* 102, 133, 1981.
62. Brooks, A. P. and Paulley, J. W., Eosinophilic gastroenteritis: an unusual cause of vomiting, *Practitioner,* 226, 1803, 1982.
63. Cello, J. P., Eosinophilic gastroenteritis, *Am. J. Med.,* 67, 1097, 1979.
64. Klein, N. C., Hargrove, L., Sleisenger, M. H., and Jeffries, G. H., Eosinophilic gastroenteritis, *Medicine (Baltimore),* 49, 299, 1970.
65. Caldwell, J. G., Tennebaum, J., and Bronstein, H. A., Serum IgE in eosinophilic gastroenteritis: response to intestinal challenge in 2 cases, *N. Engl. J. Med.,* 292, 1388, 1975.
66. Venge, P., Dahl, R., Hallgren, R., and Olsson, I., Cationic proteins of human eosinophils and their role in the inflammatory reaction, in *The Eosinophil in Health and Disease,* Mahmoud, A. A. F. and Austen, K. F., Eds., Grune & Stratton, New York, 1980, 131.
67. McLaren, D. J., McKeen, J. R., Olsson, I., Venge, P., and Kay, A. B., Morphological studies on the killing of Schistosomula of *Schistosoma mansonii* by human eosinophil and neutrophil cationic proteins in-vitro, *Parasite Immunol.,* 3, 359, 1981.
68. Capron, M., Capron A., and DeSaint, J., FC receptors for IgE on human and rat eosinophils, *J. Immunol.,* 126, 2087, 1981.
69. Tai, P. C. and Spry, C. F. J., The mechanisms which produce vacuolated and degranulated eosinophils, *Br. J. Haematol.,* 449, 219, 1981.
70. Frazer, A. C., Fletcher, R. F., and Ross, C. A. C., Gluten induced enteropathy. The effect of partially digested gluten, *Lancet,* ii, 252, 1959.
71. Ferguson, A. and Murray, D., Quantitation of intraepithelial lymphocytes in human jejunum, *Gut,* 12, 988, 1971.
72. Ferguson, A., Lymphocytes in coeliac disease, in *Coeliac Disease,* Hekkens, W. T. J. M. and Pena, A. S., Eds., Stenfert Kroese, Leiden, 1974, 135.
73. Holmes, G. K. T., Asquith, P., Stokes, P. L., and Cooke, W. T., Cellular infiltrate of jejunal biopsies in adult coeliac disease in relation to gluten withdrawal, *Gut,* 15, 278, 1974.
74. Lancaster-Smith, M., Kumar, P. J., and Dawson, A. M., The cellular infiltrate of the jejunum in adult coeliac disease and dermatitis herpetiformis following the reintroduction of dietary gluten, *Gut,* 16, 683, 1975.
75. Ferguson, A. and Parrott, D. M. U., The effect of antigen deprivation on thymus dependent and thymus independent lymphocytes in the small intestine of the mouse, *Clin. Exp. Immunol.,* 12, 477, 1972.
76. Arnaud-Battandier, F., Bundy, B. H., and O'Neill, M., Cytotoxic activities of gut mucosal lymphoid cells in guinea pigs, *J. Immunol.,* 121, 1059, 1978.
77. Adlersberg, D., Colcherand, H., and Drachman, S. R., Studies on the effects of cortisone and pituitary adreno-corticotrophic hormone on the sprue syndrome, *Gastroenterology,* 19, 674, 1951.
78. Cooke, W. T., The effect of corticotrophin in idiopathic steatorrhoea, *Lancet,* 2, 425, 1953.
79. Wall, A. J., Douglas, A. P., Booth, C. C. and Pearse, A. G. E., Response of the jejunal mucosa in adult coeliac disease to oral prednisolone, *Gut,* 11, 7, 1970.
80. Falchuk, Z. M. and Katz, A. J., Organ culture model of gluten-sensitive enteropathy, in *Perspectives in Coeliac Disease,* McNicholl, B., McCarthy, C. F., and Fottrell, P. F., Eds., MTP Press, Lancaster, 1978, 65.
81. Katz, A. J., Falchuk, Z. M., Strober, W., and Shwachman, H., Gluten sensitive enteropathy. Inhibition by cortisol of the effect of gluten protein in-vitro, *N. Engl. J. Med.,* 295, 131, 1976.
82. Asquith, P., Immunology of coeliac disease, *Clin. Gastroenterol.,* 3, 213, 1974.
83. Asquith, P., Thompson, R. A., and Cooke, W. T., Serum immunoglobulins in adult coeliac disease, *Lancet,* 2, 129, 1969.
84. Hobbs, J. R. and Hepner, G. W., Deficiency of gamma M globulin in coeliac disease, *Lancet,* I, 217, 1968.
85. Baklein, K., Brandtzaeg, P., and Fausa, O., Immunoglobulins in jejunal mucosa and serum from patients with adult coeliac disease, *Scand. J. Gastroenterol.,* 12, 149, 1977.
86. Asquith, P., Housley, J., and Cooke, W. T., Serum and intestinal immunoglobulins in adult coeliac disease, in *Coeliac Disease,* Booth, C. C. and Dowling R. H., Eds., Churchill Livingstone, Edinburgh, 1970, 151.
87. Thompson, R. A., Asquith, P., and Cooke, W. T., Secretory IgA in the serum, *Lancet,* 2, 517, 1969.
88. Kendrick, K. G. and Walker-Smith, J. A., Immunoglobulins and dietary protein antibodies in childhood coeliac disease, *Gut,* 11, 635, 1970.
89. Ferguson, A. and Carswell, F., Precipitins to dietary proteins in serum and upper intestinal secretions of coeliac children, *Br. Med. J.,* 1, 75, 1972.

90. Katz, J., Kantor, F. S., and Herskovic, T., Intestinal antibodies to wheat fractions in coeliac disease, *Ann. Intern. Med.*, 69, 1149, 1968.
91. Stern, M., Fischer, K., and Gruttner, R., Immunofluorescent serum gliadin antibodies in children with coeliac disease and various malabsorptive disorders, *Eur. J. Paediatr.*, 130, 155, 1979.
92. Savilahti, E., Perkkio, M., Kalimo, K., Viander, M., Vainio, E., and Reunala, T., IgA antigliadin antibodies: a marker of mucosal damage in childhood coeliac disease, *Lancet*, i, 320, 1981.
93. Unsworth, D. J., Kieffer, M., Holborow, E. J., Coombs, R. R. A., and Walker-Smith, J. A., IgA antigliadin antibodies in coeliac disease, *Clin. Exp. Immunol.*, 46, 286, 1981.
94. Kendall, J. J., Cox, P. S., Schneider, R., and Hawkins, C. F., Gluten subfractions in coeliac disease, *Lancet*, ii, 1065, 1972.
95. Howdle, P. D., Ciclitira, P. J., Simpson, F. G., and Losowsky, M. S., Are all gliadins toxic in coeliac disease?, *Gut*, 22, 874, 1981.
96. O'Farrelly, C., Kelly, J., Hekkens, W., Bradley, B., Thompson, A., Feighery, C., and Weir, D. G., Alpha gliadin antibody levels: a serological test for coeliac disease, *Br. Med. J.*, 286, 2007, 1983.
97. Haeney, M. R. and Asquith, P., Inhibition of leucocyte migration by alpha gliadin in patients with gastrointestinal disease: its specificity with respect to coeliac disease and alpha gliadin, in *Perspectives in Coeliac Disease*, McNicholl, B., McCarthy, C. F., and Fottrell, P. F., Eds., MTP Press, Lancaster, 1978, 229.
98. O'Farrelly, C., Feighery, C., Greally, J., and Weir, D. G., Cellular response to alpha gliadin in untreated coeliac disease, *Gut*, 23, 83, 1983.
99. O'Farrelly, C., Whelan, C. A., Feighery, C. F., and Weir, D. G., Coeliac mononuclear cells bind alpha gliadin monoclonal antibody, in press.
100. Doe, W., Booth, C. C., and Brown, D. L., Evidence for complement binding immune complexes in adult coeliac disease, Crohn's disease and ulcerative colitis, *Lancet*, i, 402, 1973.
101. Theofilopoulous, A. N. and Dixon, F. J., The biology and detection of immune complexes, *Adv. Immunol.*, 28, 89, 1979.
102. Bullen, A. W., Maini, R. N., and Losowsky, M. S., Circulating immune complexes in coeliac disease, *Gut*, 21, 915, 1980.
103. Hall, R. P., Strober, W., Katz, S. I., and Lawley, T. J., IgA containing circulating immune complexes in gluten sensitive enteropathy, *Clin. Exp. Immunol.*, 45, 234, 1981.
104. Corazza, G. R., Lazzari, R., Londei, M., Frisoni, M., Collina, A., and Gasbarrini, G., CIq binding activity in childhood coeliac disease, *Int. J. Gastroenterol.*, 15, 14, 1983.
105. Paganelli, R., Levinsky, R. J., Brostoff, J., and Wraith, D. G., Immune complexes containing food proteins in normal and atopic subjects after oral challenge and effect of sodium cromoglycate on antigen absorption, *Lancet*, 1, 1270, 1979.
106. Seah, P. P., Fry, L., Hoffbrand, A. V., and Holborow, E. J., Tissue antibodies in dermatitis herpetiformis and adult coeliac disease, *Lancet*, i, 834, 1971.
107. Alp, M. H. and Wright, R., Autoantibodies to reticulin in patients with idiopathic steatorrhoea, coeliac disease and Crohn's disease and their relation to immunoglobulins and dietary antibodies, *Lancet*, 2, 682, 1971.
108. Seah, P. P., Fry, L., Holborow, E. J., Rossiter, M. A., Doe, W. F., Magalhaes, A. G., and Hoffbrand, A. V., Antireticulin antibody: incidence and diagnostic significance, *Gut*, 14, 311, 1973.
109. Magalhaes, A. G. N., Peters, T. J., and Doe, W. F., Studies on the nature and significance of connective tissue antibodies in adult coeliac disease and Crohn's disease, *Gut*, 15, 284, 1974.
110. Eade, O. E., Lloyd, R. S., Lang, C., and Wright, R., IgA and IgG reticulin antibodies in coeliac disease and non-coeliac patients, *Gut*, 18, 991, 1977.
111. Mawhinney, H. and Love, A. H. G., Antireticulin antibody in jejunal juice in coeliac disease, *Clin. Exp. Immunol.*, 21, 394, 1975.
112. Williamson, N., Asquith, P., Stokes, P. L., Jowett, A. W., and Cooke, W. T., Anticonnective tissue and other antitissue 'antibodies' in the sera of patients with coeliac disease compared with the findings in a mixed hospital population, *J. Clin. Pathol.*, 29, 484, 1976.
113. Loeb, P. M. Strober, W., and Falchuk, Z., Incorporation of leucine-14c into immunoglobulins by jejunal biopsies of the patients with coeliac sprue and other gastrointestinal disease, *J. Clin. Invest.*, 50, 559, 1971.
114. Falchuk, Z. M. and Strober W., Gluten sensitive enteropathy; synthesis of antigliadin antibody in-vitro, *Gut*, 15, 947, 1974.
115. Brandtzaeg, P. and Baklein, K., Immunohistochemical studies of the formation and epithelial transport of immunoglobulins in normal and diseased human intestinal mucosa, *Scand. J. Gastroenterol.*, 11, 5, 1976.
116. Shiner, M. and Ballard, J., Antigen-antibody reactions in jejunal mucosa in childhood coeliac disease after gluten challenge, *Lancet*, I, 1202, 1972.
117. Scott, B. B., Boodall, A., Stephenson, P. M., and Jenkins, D., Is reaginic hypersensitivity involved in coeliac disease? *Gut*, 24 (Abstr F33), 1983.

118. McLaughlin, P., Hunter, J. O., Easter, G. B., Alun-Jones, V., Calladine, M. R H., and Coombs, R. R. A., Histamine release, in-vitro, from the jejunal mucosa following challenge with gliadin and also anti-IgE, in *Proc. 2nd Fisions Food Allergy Workshop,* Medicine Publishing Foundation, Oxford, 1983, 7.
119. Williams, A., Asquith, P., and Stableforth, D., Asthma, eczema, seasonal rhinitis and skin atopy in adult coeliac disease, *Gut,* 25, A151, 1984.
120. Webster, A. D. B., Slavin, G., Shiner, M., Platta-Mills, T., and Asherson, G. L., Coeliac disease with severe hypogammaglobulinaemia, *Gut,* 22, 153, 1981.
121. Marsh, M. N. and Haeney, M. R., Studies of intestinal lymphoid tissue. VI. Proliferative response of small intestinal epithelial lymphocytes distinguishes gluten from non-gluten-induced enteropathy, *J. Clin. Pathol.,* 36, 149, 1983.
122. Douwes, F. R., Gluten and lymphocyte sensitisation in coeliac disease, *Lancet,* 2, 1353, 1976.
123. Haeney, M. R. and Asquith, P., Inhibition of leucocyte migration by alpha gliadin in patients with gastrointestinal disease: its specificity with respect to alpha gliadin and coeliac disease, in *Perspectives in Coeliac Disease,* McNicholl, B., McCarthy, C. F., and Fottrell, P. F., Eds., MTP Press, Lancaster, 1978, 155.
124. Bullen, A. W. and Losowsky, M. S., Cell mediated immunity to gluten fraction III in adult coeliac disease, *Gut,* 19, 126, 1978.
125. Ashkenazi, A., Idar, D., Barzitai, N., Leven, S., Or, A., and Handzel, Z. T., Effect of gluten-free diet on an immunological assay for coeliac disease, *Lancet,* 914, 1981.
126. O'Farrelly, C., Feighery, C., Greally, J. F., and Weir, D. G., Cellular response to alpha-gliadin in untreated coeliac disease, *Gut,* 23, 83, 1983.
127. Simpson, F. G., Bullen, A. W., Robertson, D. A. F., and Losowsky, M. F., HLA-B8 and cell mediated immunity to gluten, *Gut,* 22, 633, 1981.
128. Simpson, F. G., Field, H. P., Howdle, P. D., Robertson, D. A. F., and Losowsky, M. F., Leucocyte migration inhibition test in coeliac disease — a reappraisal, *Gut,* 23, 311, 1983.
129. Ansaldi, N., De Sanctis, C., Fabris, C., and Ponzone, A., Blastizzone linfocitaria in-vitro con fitemoglutinina E con glutine inbambina affeti da morbo celiaco, *Minerva Paediatr.,* 22, 1907, 1979.
130. Morganroth, J., Watson, D. W., and French, A. B., Cellular and humoral sensitivity to gluten fractions in patients with treated non-tropical sprue, *Am. J. Dig. Dis.,* 17, 205, 1972.
131. Holmes, G. K. T., Asquith, P., and Cooke, W. T., Cell mediated immunity to gluten fraction III in adult coeliac disease, *Clin. Exp. Immunol.,* 24, 259, 1976.
132. Selby, W. S., Janossy, G., Bofill, M., and Jewell, D. P., Lymphocyte subpopulations in the human small intestine. The findings in normal mucosa and in the mucosa of patients with adult coeliac disease, *Clin. Exp. Immunol.,* 52, 219, 1983.
133. Marsh, M. N., Studies of intestinal lymphoid tissue. III. Quantitative analyses of epithelial lymphocytes in the small intestine of human control subjects and of patients with coeliac sprue, *Gastroenterology,* 79, 481, 1980.
134. Marsh, M. N., Abnormal behaviour of epithelial lymphocytes in sprue, *Gastroenterology,* 78, 1218, 1980.
135. Marsh, M. N., Studies of intestinal lymphoid tissue. V. The cytology and electron microscopy of gluten-sensitive enteropathy, with particular reference to its immunopathology, *Scand. J. Gastroenterol.,* 16 (Suppl. 70), 87, 1981.
136. Marsh, M. N. and Haeney, M. R., Studies of intestinal lymphoid tissue. VI. Proliferative response of small intestinal epithelial lymphocytes distinguishes gluten from non-gluten-induced enteropathy, *J. Clin. Pathol.,* 36, 149, 1983.
137. Ferguson, A. and Jarrett, E. E. E., Hypersensitivity reactions in the small intestine. I. Thymus dependence of experimental partial villous atrophy, *Gut,* 16, 114, 1975.
138. MacDonald, T. T. and Ferguson, A., Effects of allograft rejection on mucosal architecture and lymphoid cell infiltrate, *Gut,* 17, 81, 1976.
139. MacDonald, T. T. and Ferguson, A., The effects of allograft rejection and graft-versus host disease on epithelial cell kinetics, *Cell Tissue Kinet.,* 10, 301, 1977.
140. Ferguson, A., McClure, J. P., MacDonald, T. T., and Holden, R. J., Cell mediated immunity to gliadin within the small intestinal mucosa in coeliac disease, *Lancet,* i, 895, 1975.
141. Asquith, P., Immunology, *Clin. Gastroenterol.,* 3, 213, 1974.
142. Baker, P. G. and Read, A. E., Positive skin reactions to gluten in coeliac disease, *Q. J. Med.,* 45, 603, 1976.
143. Rawcliffe, P. M., Anand, B. S., Offord, R. E., Piris, J., and Truelove, S. C., A skin test for coeliac disease, in *Perspective in Coeliac Disease,* McNicholl, B., McCarthy, C. F., and Fottrell, P. F., Eds., MTP Press, Lancaster, 1978, 347.
144. Stokes, P. L., Ferguson, A., Holmes, G. K. T., and Cooke, W. T., Familial aspects of coeliac disease, *Q. J. Med.,* 45, 567, 1976.

145. Stokes, P. L., Asquith P., Holmes, G. K. T., Mackintosh, P., and Cooke, W. T., Histocompatibility antigens associated with adult coeliac disease, *Lancet*, 2, 162, 1972.
146. Falchuk, Z. M., Rogentine, G. N., and Strober, W., Predominance of histocompatibility antigen HL-A8 in patients with gluten sensitive enteropathy, *J. Clin. Invest.*, 51, 1602, 1972.
147. Keuning, J. J., Pena, A. S., Van-Leeuwen, A., Van Hooff, J. P., and Van Rood, J. J., HLA-DW3 associated with coeliac disease, *Lancet*, I, 506, 1976.
148. Betuel, H., Gebuhrer, L., D'Scos, L., Percebois, H., Minaire, Y., and Betrand, J., Adult coeliac disease associated with HLA-DRW3, and DRW7 *Tissue Antigens*, 15, 231, 1980.
149. Mann, D. D. L., Katz, S. I., Nelson, D. L., Abelson, L. D., and Strober, W., Specific B-cell antigens associated with gluten-sensitive enteropathy and dermatitis herpetiformis, *Lancet*, i, 110, 1976.
150. Pena, A. S., Mann, D. L., Hague, N. E., Heck, J. A., Van Leeuwen, A., Van Rood, J. J., and Strober, W., Genetic basis of gluten sensitive enteropathy, *Gastroenterology*, 15, 230, 1978.
151. Kagnoff, M. F., Two genetic loci control the murine immune response to A-gliadin, a wheat protein that activates coeliac sprue, *Nature*, 296, 158, 1982.
152. Tosi, R., Vismara, D., Tanigaki, N., Ferara, G. B., Cicimarra, F., Buffolano, W., Follo, D., and Auricchio, S., Evidence that coeliac disease is primarily associated with a DC locus allelic specificity, *Clin. Immunol. Immunopathol.*, 28, 395, 1983.
153. Elliott, E. J., Sachs, J. A., Awad, J., Naverete, C., and Walker-Smith, J. A., Histocompatibility antigens and clinical features in coeliac disease, *Gut*, 25, 10. 1984.
154. Strober, W., Falchuk, Z. M., and Rogentine, G. N., The pathogenesis of gluten sensitive enteropathy, *Ann. Intern. Med.*, 83, 242, 1975.
155. Rubin, W., Fauci, A. S., and Sleisenger, M. H., Immunofluorescent studies in adult coeliac disease, *J. Clin. Invest.*, 44, 475, 1965.
156. Douglas, A. P., The binding of glycopeptide component of wheat gluten to intestinal mucosa of normal and coeliac human subjects, *Clin. Chim. Acta*, 73, 357, 1976.
157. Stern, M., Dietrich, R., and Gruttner, R., Gliadin binding immunocytes in small intestinal lamina propria of children with coeliac disease, *Paediatr. Res.*, 15, 1196, 1981.
158. Ciclitira, P. J., Ellis, H. J., Wood, G. M., Howdle, P. D., and Losowsky, M. S., Gliadin antibody secretion by coeliac jejunal mucosa, *Gut*, 25, 10, 1984.
159. Doe, W. F., Henry, K., and Booth, C. C., Complement in coeliac disease in *Coeliac Disease*, Hekkens, W. T. J. M. and Pena, A. S., Eds., Stenfert Kroese, Leiden, 1974, 189.
160. Shiner, M., Ultrastructural changes suggestive of immune reactions in the jejunal mucosa of coeliac children following gluten challenge, *Gut*, 14, 1, 1973.
161. Cunningham-Rundles, S., Cunningham-Rundles, C., and Pollack, M. S., Response to wheat antigen in in-vitro lymphocyte transformation among HLA-B8 positive normal donors, *Transplant. Proc.*, 10, 977, 1978.
162. Falchuk, Z. M., Gluten sensitive enteropathy, in *Malabsorption and Nutritional Support*, Sleisenger, M. H., Ed., W. B. Saunders, London, 1983, 475.
163. Weisar, M. M. and Douglas, A. P., An alternative mechanism for gluten toxicity in coeliac disease, *Lancet*, i, 567, 1976.
164. Lorenson, V. and Olsen, W. A., In-vivo responses of rat intestinal epithelium to intralumenal dietary lectins, *Gastroenterology*, 83, 838, 1982.
165. Kottgen, E., Volk, B., Kluge, F., and Gerok, W., Gluten, a lectin with oligomannosyl specificity and the causative agent of gluten-sensitive enteropathy, *Biochem. Biophys. Res. Commun.*, 109, 168, 1982.
166. Kuitunen, P., Visakorpi, J. K., Savilahti, E., and Pelkonen, P., Malabsorption syndrome with cows milk intolerance, *Arch. Dis. Child.* 50, 351, 1975.
167. Goldman, A. S., Anderson, D. W., Sellers, W. A., Saperstein, S., Knicker, W. T., and Halpern, S. R., Milk allergy. I. Oral challenge with milk and isolated milk proteins in allergic children, *Paediatrics*, 32, 425, 1963.
168. Frier, S. and Kletter, B., Milk allergy in infants and young children, *Clin. Paediatr.*, 9, 449, 1970.
169. Gerrard, J. W., MacKenzie, J. W. A., Goluboff, N., Garsson, J. Z., and Maningas, C. S., Cows milk allergy: prevalence and manifestations in an unselected series of newborns, *Acta Paediatr. Scand.*, 234, 1, 1973.
170. Bahna, S. L. and Gandhi, M., Milk hypersensitivity. I. Pathogenesis and symptomatology, *Ann. Allergy*, 50(4), 218, 1983.
171. Jenkins, H. R., Picutt, J. R., Soothill, J. F., Milla, P. J., and Harries, J. T., Food allergy: the major cause of infantile colitis, *Arch. Dis. Child.*, 59(4), 326, 1984.
172. Whorwell, P. J., Holdstock, G., Whorwell, G. M., and Wright, R., Bottle feeding, early gastroenteritis and inflammatory bowel disease, *Br. Med. J.*, i, 382, 1979.
173. Walker-Smith, J. A., Cows milk intolerance, in *Topics in Gastroenterology*, Vol. 10, Jewell, D. P. and Selby, W. S., Eds., Blackwell Scientific, Oxford, 1982, 257.

174. DePayer, E. and Walker-Smith, J. A., Cows milk intolerance presenting as necrotising enterocolitis, *Helvetica Paediatr. Acta.*, 32, 509, 1977.
175. Parrish, W. E., Barrett, A. M., Coombs, R. R. A., Gunther, M., and Camps, F. E., Hypersensitivity to milk and sudden death in infancy, *Lancet*, ii, 1106, 1969.
176. Devey, M. E., Anderson, K. J., Coombs, R. R. A., Henschel, M. J., and Coates, M. E., The modified anaphylaxis hypothesis for cot death: anaphylactic sensitization in guinea pigs fed cows milk, *Clin. Exp. Immunol.*, 26, 542, 1976.
177. McLaughlin, P. and Coombs, R. R. A., Latent anaphylactic sensitivity of infants to cows milk proteins: histamine release from blood basophils, *Clin. Allergy*, 13, 1983.
178. Gerrard, J. W. and Shenassa, M., Sensitization to substances in breast milk: recognition, management and significance, *Ann. Allergy*, 51, 300, 1983.
179. May, C. D., Fomon, G., and Remigio, A., Immunologic consequences of feeding children with cow milk and soya products, *Acta Paediatr. Scand.*, 71, 43, 1982.
180. Gunther, M., Aschaffenberg, R., Matthews, R. H., Parrish, W. E., and Coombs, R. R. A., The level of antibodies to the proteins of cows milk in the serum of normal human infants, *Immunology*, 3, 296, 1960.
181. Shiner, M., Ballard, J., and Smith, M. E., The small intestinal mucosa in cows milk allergy, *Lancet*, i, 136, 1975.
182. Jackson, D., Phillips, A. D., Haidas, A., and Walker-Smith, J. A., Morphological studies of the small intestine in children with food intolerance and related problems in *Proc. 2nd Fisons Food Allergy Workshop*, Coombs, R. R. A., Ed., Medicine Publishing, Foundation, Oxford, 1983, 10.
183. Cunningham-Rundles, C., Brandeis, W. E., Good, R. A., and Day, N. K., Milk precipitins, circulating immune complexes and IgA deficiency, *Proc. Natl. Acad. Sci. U.S.A.*, 75, 3387, 1978.
184. Dannaeus, A. and Johansson, S. G. O., A follow up study of infants with adverse reactions to cows milk. I. Serum IgE, skin test reactions and RAST in relation to clinical course, *Acta Paediatr. Scand.*, 68, 377, 1979.
185. Ford, P. K., Hill, D. J., and Hosking, C. S., Cows milk hypersensitivity: immediate and delayed onset of clinical patterns, *Arch. Dis. Child.*, 11, 856, 1983.
186. Rosekrans, P. C. M., Meijer, C. J. L. M., Cornelisse, C. J., Vanderwal, A. M., and Lindeman, J., Use of morphometry and immunochemistry of small intestinal biopsy specimens in the diagnosis of food allergy, *J. Clin. Pathol.*, 33, 25, 1980.
187. Pearson, J. R., Antibody production to milk proteins in the jejunal mucosa of children with cows milk protein intolerance, *Paediatr. Res.*, 17, 406, 1983.
188. Deline, M., Cambiaso, C., and Masson, P. L., Circulating immune complexes in infants fed on cows milk, *Nature*, 272, 632, 1978.
189. Frick, O. L., β-Lactoglobulin in immune complexes in milk sensitive children, *J. Allergy Clin. Immunol.*, 69 (Suppl.), 157, 1982.
190. Paganelli, R., Atherton, D. J., and Levinsky, J., Difference between normal and milk allergic subjects in their immune responses after milk ingestion, *Arch. Dis. Child.*, 58, 201, 1983.
191. Firer, M. A., Cows milk allergy and eczema: patterns of the antibody response to cows milk in allergic skin disease, *Clin. Allergy*, 12, 385, 1982.
192. Fontaine, J. L. and Navarro, J., Small intestinal biopsy in cows milk protein allergy in infancy, *Arch. Dis. Child.*, 50, 357, 1975.
193. Scheinmamm, P., Gendel, D., Charlas, J., and Pampe, J., The value of lymphoblast transformation test in cows milk protein intestinal intolerance, *Clin. Allergy*, 6, 515, 1976.
194. Minor, J. D., Tolber, S. G., and Frick, O. L., Leucocyte inhibition factor in delayed-onset food allergy, *J. Allergy Clin. Immunol.*, 66(4), 314, 1980.
195. Ferguson, A., Pathogenesis and mechanisms in the gastrointestinal tract, in *Proc. 1st Fisons Food Allergy Workshop*, Coombs, R. R. A., Ed., Medicine Publishing Foundation, Oxford, 1980, 28.
196. Verkasalu, M., Kuitunen, P., Tiilikainen, A., and Savilahti, E., HLA antigens in intestinal cows milk allergy, *Acta Paediatr. Scand.*, 72, 19, 1983.
197. Ament, M. E. and Rubin, C. E., Soya protein — another cause of the flat intestinal lesion, *Gastroenterology*, 62, 227, 1972.
198. Goel, K., Lifshitz, F., Kahn, E., and Teichberg, S., Monosaccharide intolerance and soya protein hypersensitivity in an infant with diarrhoea, *J. Paediatr.*, 93, 617, 1978.
199. Whittington, P. F. and Gibson, R., Soya protein intolerance: four patients with concomitant cows milk intolerance, *Paediatrics*, 59, 730, 1977.
200. Perkkio, M., Savilahti, E., and Kuitunen, P., Morphometric and immunohistochemical study of jejunal biopsies from children with intestinal soya allergy, *Eur. J. Paediatr.*, 137, 63, 1981.
201. Barrett, M. E. J., Strachan, P. J., and Porter, P., Antibody mechanisms implicated in the digestive disturbances following ingestion of soya protein in calves and pigs, *Clin. Exp. Immunol.*, 31, 305, 1978.

202. Butler, H. L., Byrne, W. J., Marmer, D. J., Euler, A. R., and Steele, R. W., Depressed neutrophil chemotaxis in infants with cows milk and/or soya protein intolerance, *Paediatrics,* 67, 264, 1981.
203. Bellamy, J. E. C. and Nielson, S. O., Immune mediated emigration of neutrophils into the lumen of the small intestine, *Infect. Immunol.,* 9, 615, 1974.
204. Peters, T. J., Jones, P. F., Jenkins, W. J., and Wells, G., Analytical subcellular fractionation of jejunal biopsy specimens. Enzyme activities, organelle pathology and response to cortico-steroids in patients with non-responsive coeliac disease, *Clin. Sci. Mol. Med.,* 55, 293, 1978.
205. Tongeren, J. H. M., Cluysenaer, O. J. J., and Schillings, P. H. M., Refractory sprue in *Perspectives in Coeliac Disease,* McNicholl, B., McCarthy, C. F., and Fottrell, P. F., MTP Press, Lancaster, 1978, 323.
206. Bossart, R., Henry, K., Booth, C. C., and Doe, W. F., Collagenous basement membrane thickening in jejunal biopsies from patients with adult coeliac disease, *Gut,* 15, 338, 1975.
207. Love, A. H. G., Elmes, M., Golden, M. K. and McMaster, D., Zinc deficiency and coeliac disease, in *Perspectives in Coeliac Disease,* McNicholl, B., McCarthy, C. F., and Fottrell, P. F., Eds., MTP Press, Lancaster, 1978, 335.
208. Mike, N. and Asquith, P., Soya protein hypersensitivity in non-responsive coeliac disease, *Gut,* 25, 10, 1984.
209. Haeney, M. R., Goodwin, B. J. F., Barrett, M. E. J., Mike, N., and Asquith, P., Soya protein antibodies in man: their occurrence and possible relevance in coeliac disease, *J. Clin. Pathol.,* 35, 319, 1982.
210. Mike, N., Haeney, M. R., and Asquith, P., Cell mediated immunity to soya protein in coeliac disease, *Gut,* 24, 10, 1983.
211. Mayberry, J. F., Rhodes, J., and Newcombe, R. G., Familial prevalence of inflammatory bowel disease in relatives of patients with Crohn's disease, *Br. Med. J.,* 1, 84, 1980.
212. Edwards, F. C. and Truelove, S. C., Course and prognosis of ulcerative colitis, *Gut,* 5, 1, 1964.
213. Alarcon-Segovia, D., Herskovic, T., Dearing, W. H., Bartholomew, L. H., Cain, J. C., and Shorter, R. G., Lupus erythematosis cell phenomenon in patients with chronic ulcerative colitis, *Gut,* 6, 39, 1965.
214. Wright, R. S. and Truelove, S. C., Autoimmune reactions in ulcerative colitis, *Gut,* 7, 32, 1966.
215. O'Morain, C., Jaegar, R., and Das, K. M., Possible role for anti-idiotypic antibodies in Crohn's disease, *Gut,* 25, 10, 1984.
216. Stocker, W., Otte, M., Normann, D., Ulrich, S., and Dageford, J., Autoantibodies to pancreatic acini and to intestinal goblet cells in patients with Crohn's disease and ulcerative colitis, paper presented at 12th Int. Congr. Gastroenterol., Lisbon, September 1984, 87.
217. Hodgson, H. J. F., Potter, B. J., and Jewell, D. P., Immune complexes in ulcerative colitis and Crohn's disease, *Clin. Exp. Immunol.,* 29, 187, 1977.
218. Kirk, B. W. and Freedman, S. O., Hypogammaglobulinaemia, thymoma and ulcerative colitis, *Can. Med. Assoc. J.,* 96, 1272, 1967.
219. Hodgson, H. J. F. and Jewell, D. P., The humoral immune system in inflammatory bowel disease, *Am. J. Dig. Dis.,* 23, 123, 1978.
220. Thompson, R. A., Asquith, P., and Cooke, W. T., Secretory IgA in the serum, *Lancet,* ii, 517, 1969.
221. Bendixen, G., Goltermann, N., Tarnum, S., Jensen, K. B., Weeke, B., and Westergaard, H., Immunoglobulin and albumin turnover in ulcerative colitis, *Scand. J. Gastroenterol.,* 5, 433, 1970.
222. Hodgson, H. J. F., Potter, B. J., and Jewell, D. P., C3 metabolism in ulcerative colitis and Crohn's disease, *Clin. Exp. Immunol.,* 28, 490, 1977.
223. Auer, I. O., Gotz, S., Ziemer, E., Malchow, J., and Ehms, H., Immune status in Crohn's disease. II. Peripheral blood B lymphocytes enumerated by means of F(AB)2 antibody fragments, null and T lymphocytes, *Gut,* 20, 261, 1979.
224. Roche, J. K., Watkins, M. H., and Cook, S. L., Inflammatory bowel disease: prevalence and level of activation of circulating T lymphocyte subpopulations mediating suppressor/cytotoxic and helper function as defined by monoclonal antibodies, *Clin. Immunol. Immunopathol.,* 25, 362, 1981.
225. Strickland, R. G., Korsmeyer, S., Soltis, R. D., Wilson, I. D., and Williams, R. C., Peripheral blood T and B cells in chronic inflammatory bowel disease, *Gastroenterology,* 67, 569, 1974.
226. Sieber, G., Herrmann, F., Zeitz, M., Teichmann, H., and Ruhl, H., Abnormalities of B cell activation and immunoregulation in patients with Crohn's disease, *Gut,* 25 1255, 1984.
227. Williams, W. J., A study of Crohn's syndrome using tissue extracts and the Kvein and Mantux tests, *Gut,* 6, 503, 1965.
228. Morgenroth, J. and Watson, D. W., Sensitivity to atypical mycobacterial antigens in patients with Crohn's disease, *Am. J. Dig. Dis.,* 15, 653, 1970.
229. Meuwissen, S. G. M., Schellekens, P., Th, A., Huismans, L., and Tytgat, G. V., Impaired anamnestic cellular immune response in patients with Crohn's disease, *Gut,* 16, 854, 1975.
230. Ainley, C. C., Cason, J., Wolstencroft, P. W., Keeling, N., and Thompson, R. P. H., Abnormal cell mediated immunity in inflammatory bowel disease, *Gut,* 25, 10, 1984.

231. Sachar, D. B., Taub, R. N., Brown, S. M., Present, D. H., Korelitz, B. I., and Janowitz, H. D., Impaired lymphocyte responsiveness in inflammatory bowel disease, *Gastroenterology*, 64, 203, 1973.
232. Brown, S. M., Taub, R. N., Present, D. H., and Janowitz, H. D., Short-term lymphocyte cultures in regional enteritis, *Lancet*, i, 1112, 1970.
233. Bird, A. G. and Britton, S., No evidence for decreased lymphocyte reactivity in Crohn's disease, *Gastroenterology*, 67, 926, 1974.
234. Ainley, C. C., Cason, J., Slavin, B. M., Wolstencroft, R. A., Keeling, P. W. N., and Thompson, R. P. H., Malnutrition, but not zinc deficiency, causes depressed cell mediated immunity in Crohn's disease, *Gut*, 25, 10, 1984.
235. Kelleher, D., Murphy, A., Feighery, C., Whelan, C. A., Keeling, P. W. N., and Weir, D. G., Lymphocyte transformation in inflammatory bowel disease — effect of monocyte suppressor cell, *Gut*, 25, 10, 1984.
236. Selby, W. S. and Jewell, D. P., T lymphocyte subsets in inflammatory bowel disease: peripheral blood, *Gut*, 24, 99, 1983.
237. Makiyama, K., Selby, W. S., and Jewell, D. P., E rosetting lymphocytes in inflammatory bowel disease. An analysis using monoclonal antibody, *Clin. Exp. Immunol.*, 52, 350, 1983.
238. Godin, N. J., Sachar, D. B., Winchester, R., Simon, C., and Janowitz, H. D., Loss of suppressor T cells in active inflammatory bowel disease, *Gut*, 25, 743, 1984.
239. Victorino, R. M. M. and Hodgson, H. J. F., Alterations in T lymphocyte subpopulations in inflammatory bowel disease, *Clin. Exp. Immunol.*, 41, 156, 1980.
240. Holdstock, G., Chastenay, B. F., and Krawitt, E. L., Functional suppressor T cell activity in Crohn's disease and the effects of sulphasalazine, *Clin. Exp. Immunol.*, 48, 619, 1982.
241. Elson, C. O., Braeff, A. S., James, S. P., and Strober, W., Covert suppressor T cells in Crohn's disease, *Gastroenterology*, 80, 1513, 1981.
242. Meuwissen, S. G. M., Feltkamp-Vroom, T. M., de la Riviere, A. B., Von Dem Borne, A. E. G., and Tytgat, G. N., Analysis of the lympho-plasmacytic infiltrate in Crohn's disease with special reference to the identification of lymphocyte subpopulations, *Gut*, 17, 770, 1976.
243. Baklien, K. and Brandtzaeg, P., Comparative mapping of the local distribution of immunoglobulin-containing cells in ulcerative colitis and Crohn's disease, *Clin. Exp. Immunol.*, 22, 197, 1975.
244. Brandtzaeg, P. and Baklein, K., Immunohistochemical studies of the formation and epithelial transportation of immunoglobulins in normal and diseased human intestinal mucosa, *Scand. J. Gastroenterol.*, 11, 1, 1976.
245. Von Spreeuwel, J. P., Lindeman, J., Van Der Wal, A. M., Weterman, I., Kreuning, J., and Meijer, C. J. L. M., Morphological and immunohistochemical findings in upper gastrointestinal biopsies of patients with Crohn's disease of the ileum and colon, *J. Clin. Pathol.*, 35, 934, 1982.
246. Bertone, A. and Guidetti, C. S., Distribution of immunoglobulin containing cells in rectal biopsies from patients with IBD, paper presented at 12th Int. Congr. Gastroenterol., Lisbon, September 1984.
247. Bookman, M. A. and Bull, D. M., Characteristics of isolated intestinal mucosal lymphoid cells in inflammatory bowel disease, *Gastroenterology*, 77, 503, 1979.
248. MacDermott, R. P., Nash, G. S., Bertovich, M. J., Seiden, M. V., Bragdon, M. J., and Beale, M. G., Alterations of IgM, IgG and IgA synthesis and secretion by peripheral and intestinal mononuclear cells from patients with ulcerative colitis and Crohn's disease, *Gastroenterology*, 81, 844, 1981.
249. Verspaget, H., Weterman, I., and Pena, S., Immunoglobulin synthesis by intestinal and peripheral blood lymphocytes in Crohn's disease, paper presented at 12th Int. Congr. Gastroenterol., Lisbon, September 1984, 282.
250. Strickland, R. G., Husby, G., Black, W. C., and Williams, R. C., Peripheral blood and intestinal lymphocyte subpopulations in Crohn's disease, *Gut*, 16, 847, 1975.
251. Selby W. S., Janossy, G., Bofill, M., and Jewell, D. P., in *Topics in Gastroenterology*, Vol. 2, Jewell, D. P. and Shepherd, H. A., Eds., Blackwell Scientific, Oxford, 1983, 307.
252. Shorter, R. G., Tg cells and non-specific concanavalin-A induced suppressor cell activity in vitro in colonic inflammatory bowel disease and in colorectal carcinoma, in *Recent Advances in Crohn's Disease*, Pena, A. S., Weterman, I. T., Booth, C. C., and Strober, W., Eds., Martinus-Nijhoff, The Hague, 1981, 448.
253. Fiocchi, C., Battisto, J. R., and Farmer, R. G., Gut mucosal lymphocytes in inflammatory bowel disease. Isolation and preliminary functional characterization, *Dig. Dis. Sci.*, 24, 705, 1979.
254. Goodacre, R. L. and Bienenstock, J., Reduced suppressor cell activity in intestinal lymphocytes from patients with Crohn's disease, *Gastroenterology*, 82, 653, 1982.
255. Fiocchi, C., Youngman, K. R., and Farmer, R. G., Immunoregulatory function of human intestinal mucosa lymphoid cells: evidence for enhanced suppressor cell activity in inflammatory bowel disease, *Gut*, 24, 692, 1981.
256. Falchuk, Z. M., Barnhard, E., and Machado, I., Human colonic mononuclear cells (studies of cytotoxic function), *Gut*, 22, 290, 1981.

257. Gibson, P. R., Dow, E. L., Selby, W. S., Strickland, R. S., and Jewell, D. P., in *Topics in Gastroenterology*, Vol. 2, Jewell, D. P. and Shepherd, H. A., Eds., Blackwell Scientific, Oxford, 1983, 309.
258. Britton, S., Eklund, A. E., and Bird, A. G., Appearance of killer (K) cells in the mesenteric lymph nodes in Crohn's disease, *Gastroenterology*, 75, 218, 1978.
259. Meuret, G., Bitzi, A., and Hammer, B., Macrophage turnover in Crohn's disease and ulcerative colitis, *Gastroenterology*, 74, 501, 1978.
260. Whorell, P. J., Bennett, P., Tanner, A. R., and Wright, R., Monocyte function in Crohn's disease and ulcerative colitis, *Digestion*, 22, 271, 1981.
261. Mee, A. S., Szawatakowski, M., and Jewell, D. P., Monocytes in inflammatory bowel disease: phagocytosis and intracellular killing, *J. Clin. Pathol.*, 33, 921, 1980.
262. Morain, C. O., Segal, A. W., Walker, D., and Levi, A. J., Abnormalities of neutrophil function do not cause the migration effect in Crohn's disease, *Gut*, 22, 817, 1981.
263. Hermanowicz, A., Pallone, F., Gibson, P. R., and Jewell, D. P., in *Topics in Gastroenterology*, Vol. 2, Jewell, D. P. and Shepherd, H. A., Eds., Blackwell Scientific, Oxford, 1983, 307.
264. Rhodes, J. M. Potter, B. J., Brown, D. J. C., and Jewell, D. P., Serum inhibitors of leucocyte chemotaxis in Crohn's disease and ulcerative colitis, *Gastroenterology*, 82, 1327, 1982.
265. Mee, A. S. and Jewell, D. P., Monocytes in inflammatory bowel disease. Monocyte and serum lysosomal enzyme activity, *Clin. Sci.*, 58, 295, 1980.
266. Otto, H. F. and Gebbers, J. O., Electron-microscopic, ultracytochemical and immunohistological observations in Crohn's disease of the ileum and colon, *Virchows Arch.*, 391, 189, 1981.
267. Doe, W. F. and Dorsman, B., Chronic inflammatory bowel disease: increased plasminogen activator secretion by mononuclear phagocytes, *Clin. Exp. Immunol.*, 48, 256, 1982.
268. Ligumsky, M., Karmeli, F., Sharon, P., Zor, U., Cohen, F., and Rachmilewitz, F., Enhanced thromboxane A2 and prostacyclin production by cultured rectal mucosa in ulcerative colitis and its inhibition by steroids and sulphasalazine, *Gastroenterology*, 81, 444, 1981.
269. Ward, M., The pathogenesis of Crohn's disease, *Lancet*, 2, 903, 1977.
270. Gassmann, A. E. and Von Furth, R., The effect of Azathioprine on the kinetics of monocytes and macrophages during the normal steady state and an acute inflammatory reaction, *Blood*, 46, 51, 1975.
271. Rhodes, J. M. and Jewell, D. P., Inhibition of leucocyte motility by drugs used in inflammatory bowel disease, *Gut*, 22, 642, 1981.
272. Wandell, J. H. and Binder, V., Leucocyte function in Crohn's disease, *Gut*, 23, 173, 1982.
273. Ward, M. and Eastwood, M. A., The nitro blue tetrazolium test in Crohn's disease and ulcerative colitis, *Digestion*, 14, 179, 1976.
274. Kelleher, D., Feighery, C., and Weir, D. G., Neutrophil luminescence in chronic inflammatory bowel disease, *Gut*, 23, 895, 1982.
275. Verspaget, H. W., Mieremet-Ooms, M. A. C., Weterman, I. T., and Pena, A. S., Partial defect of neutrophil oxidative metabolism in Crohn's disease, *Gut*, 25, 849, 1984.
276. Lagercrantz, R., Hammarstrom, S., Perlmann, P., and Gustafsson, B. E., Immunological studies in ulcerative colitis. III. Incidence of antibodies to colon-antigen in ulcerative colitis and other gastrointestinal diseases, *Clin. Exp. Immunol.*, 1, 263, 1966.
277. Thayer, W. R., Brown, M., Sangree, M. H., Katz, J., and Hersch, T., *Escherichia coli* 0:14 and colon haemagglutinating antibodies in inflammatory bowel disease, *Gastroenterology*, 57, 311, 1969.
278. Elmgreen, J., Stahlskov, P., Permin, H., Binder, V., Heugh-Wandall, J., and Norn, S., Type I allergy to normal cellular constituents in chronic inflammatory bowel disease. Results from basophil histamine release test compared with total IgE and antinuclear antibodies, *Allergy*, 39, 17, 1984.
279. Taylor, K. B., Truelove, S. C., and Wright, R., Serologic reactions to gluten and cows milk proteins in gastrointestinal disease, *Gastroenterology*, 46, 99, 1964.
280. Falchuk, K. R. and Isselbacher, K. J., Circulating antibodies to bovine albumin in ulcerative colitis and Crohn's disease, *Gastroenterology*, 70, 5, 1976.
281. Mee, A. S., Brown, D., and Jewell, D. P., Atopy in inflammatory bowel disease, *Scand. J. Gastroenterol.*, 14, 743, 1979.
282. Jewell, D. P. and MacLennan, I. C. M., Immune complexes in inflammatory bowel disease, *Clin. Exp. Immunol.*, 14, 219, 1973.
283. Hodgson, H. J. F., Potter, B. J., and Jewell, D. P., C3 metabolism in ulcerative colitis and Crohn's disease, *Clin. Exp. Immunol.*, 28, 490, 1977.
284. McKenzie, H., Main, J., Parratt, D., and Pennington, C. R., Circulating IgA immune complexes in inflammatory bowel disease, *Gut*, 25, 10, 1984.
285. Gebbers, J. O. and Otto, H. F., Histochemical and electron microscopic observations on the local immune response in ulcerative colitis, *Virchows Arch. (Pathol. Anat.)*, 374, 271, 1977.
286. Entrican, J. H., Busuttil, A., and Ferguson, A., Histopathological features of focal lesions in the jejunal mucosa in Crohn's disease are consistent with a cell mediated immune response, *Gut*, 25, 10, 1984.

287. Fiocchi, C., Battisto, J. R., and Farmer, R. G., Studies on isolated gut mucosal lymphocytes in inflammatory bowel disease, *Dig. Dis. Sci.*, 26, 728, 1981.
288. Dykes, P. W., Delayed hypersensitivity in Crohn's disease, *Proc. R. Soc. Med.*, 63, 906, 1970.
289. Richens, E. R., Williams, M. J., Gough, K. R., and Ancill, R. J., Leucocyte migration studies in Crohn's disease using Crohn's colon homogenate and mitochondrial and microsomal fractions, *Gut*, 15, 19, 1974.
290. Bendixen, G., Cellular hypersensitivity to components of intestinal mucosa in ulcerative colitis and Crohn's disease, *Gut*, 10, 631, 1969.
291. Hunt, P. S. and Trotter, S., Lymphoblastic response to autologous colon epithelial cells in ulcerative colitis in-vitro, *Gut*, 14, 875, 1973.
292. Parent, K., Barrett, J., and Wilson, I. D., Investigation of the pathogenetic mechanisms in regional enteritis with in-vitro lymphocyte cultures, *Gastroenterology*, 61, 431, 1971.
293. Bartnik, W., Swarbrick, E. T., and Williams, C., A study of peripheral leucocyte migration in agarose-medium in inflammatory bowel disease, *Gut*, 15, 294, 1974.
294. Shorter, R. G., Cardoza, M., Spencer, R. J., and Huizenga, K. A., Further studies of in-vitro cytotoxicity of lymphocytes from patients with ulcerative and granulomatous colitis for allogeneic colonic epithelial cells, including the effects of colectomy, *Gastroenterology*, 56, 304, 1969.
295. Stobo, J. D., Tomasi, T. B., Huizenga, K. A., Spencer, R. J., and Shorter, R. G., In-vitro studies of inflammatory bowel disease. Surface receptors of the mononuclear cell required to lyse allogeneic colon epithelial cells, *Gastroenterology*, 70, 171, 1976.
296. Burnham, W. R., Gelsthorpe, K., and Langman, M. J. S., HLA-D related antigens in inflammatory bowel disease, in *Developments in Gastroenterology*, Vol. 1, Pena, A. S., Weterman, I. T., Booth, C. C., and Strober, W., Eds., Martinus-Nijhoff, The Hague, 1981, 102.
297. McConnell, R. B., Ulcerative colitis — genetic features, *Scand. J. Gastroenterol.*, 18(Suppl. 88), 14, 1982.
298. Fiasse, R., De Bruyere, M., Lantinne, D., Lienard, J. C., Willcox, R., and Dive, C., HLA-Antigens in Crohn's disease, paper presented at 12th Int. Congr. Gastroenterol., Lisbon, September 1984, 292.
299. Miller, D. S., Keighley, A. C., Smith, P. G., Hughes, A. O., and Langman, M. J. S., Crohn's disease in Nottingham: a search for time-space clustering, *Gut*, 16, 454, 1975.
300. Miller, D. S., Keighley, A. C., Smith, P. G., Hughes, A. O., and Langman, M. J. S., A case control method for seeking evidence of contagion in Crohn's disease, *Gastroenterology*, 71, 385, 1976.
301. Mayberry, J., Rhodes, J., Matthews, N., and Wensinck, F., Serum antibodies to anaerobic coccoid rods in patients with Crohn's disease or ulcerative colitis, and in medical and nursing staff, *Br. Med. J.*, 28, 108, 1981.
302. Parent, K. and Wilson, I. D., Mycobacteriophage in Crohn's disease, *Gut*, 12, 1019, 1971.
303. Persson, S., Danielsson, D., Kjellander, J., and Wallenstein, S., Studies in Crohn's disease. I. The relationship between *Yersinia enterocolitica* and terminal ileitis, *Acta Chir. Scand.*, 142, 84, 1976.
304. Elliot, P. R., Forsey, T., Darougar, S., Treharne, J. D., and Lennard-Jones, J. E., Chlamydiae and inflammatory bowel disease, *Gut*, 22, 25, 1981.
305. Gitnick, G. L., Arthur, M. H., and Shibata, I., Cultivation of viral agents from Crohn's disease, *Lancet*, 2, 215, 1976.
306. Yoshimura, H. H., Estes, M. K., and Graham, D. Y., Search for evidence of a viral aetiology for inflammatory bowel disease, *Gut*, 25, 347, 1984.
307. James, A. H., Breakfast and Crohn's disease, *Br. Med. J.*, 1, 943, 1977.
308. Rawcliffe, P. M. and Truelove, S. C., Breakfast and Crohn's disease. I, *Br. Med. J.*, 2, 539, 1978.
309. Archer, L. N. J. and Harvey, R. F., Breakfast and Crohn's disease. II, *Br. Med. J.*, 2, 540, 1978.
310. Martini, G. A. and Brandes, J. W., Increased consumption of refined carbohydrates in patients with Crohn's disease, *Klin. Wochenschr. Schu.,*, 54, 367, 1976.
311. Thornton, J. R., Emmett, P. M., and Heaton, K. W., Diet and Crohn's disease. Characteristics of the pre-illness habit, *Br. Med. J.*, 2, 762, 1979.
312. Mayberry, J. F., Rhodes, J., and Newcombe, R. B., Increased sugar consumption in Crohn's disease, *Digestion*, 20, 323, 1980.
313. Heaton, K. W., Thornton, J. R., and Emmett, P. M., Treatment of Crohn's disease with an unrefined carbohydrate, fibre rich diet, *Br. Med. J.*, 2, 764, 1979.
314. Hunter, J. O., Alun Jones, V., Freeman, A. H., Shorthouse, M., Workman, E., and McLaughlin, P., Food intolerance in gastrointestinal disorders, in Proc. 2nd Fisons Food Allergy Workshop, Coombs, R. R. A., Ed., Medicine Publishing Foundation, Oxford, 1983, 69.
315. Alun Jones, V., Dickinson, R. J., Workman, E. M., Freeman, A. H., and Hunter, J. O., Controlled trial of diet in the management of Crohn's disease, paper presented at 12th Int. Congr. Gastroenterol., Lisbon, September 1984, 943.
316. Tschaikowski, K. L., Seven years experience in allergological diagnosis and treatment of Crohn's disease, paper presented at 12th Int. Cong. Gastroenterol., Lisbon, September 1984, 497.

317. Logan, R. F. A., Edmond, M., Somerville, K. W., and Langman, M. J. S., Smoking and Crohn's disease, *Br. Med. J.*, 288, 751, 1984.
318. Farmer, R. G., Michener, W. M., and Sivak, D. S., in *Recent Advances in Crohn's Disease*, Pena A. S., Weterman, I. T., Booth, C. C., and Strober, W., Eds., Martinus-Nijhoff, The Hague, 1981, 213.
319. Lewkonia, R. M., Woodrow, J. C., McConnell, R. B., and Price-Evans, D. A., HLA-Antigens in inflammatory bowel disease, *Lancet*, i, 574, 1974.
320. Asakura, J., Tsuchiya, M., Aiso, S., Watanabe, M., Kobayashi, K., Hibi, T., Ando, K., Takata, H., and Sekiguchi, S., Association of human lymphocyte DR-2 antigen with Japanese ulceration colitis, *Gastroenterology*, 82, 413, 1980.
321. Perrett, A. D., Higgins, G., Johnston, H. H., Massarella, G. R., Truelove, S. C., and Wright, R., The liver in ulcerative colitis, *Q. J. Med.*, 40, 211, 1971.
322. Lake, A. M., Stitzel, A. E., Urmson, J. R., Walker, W. A., and Spitzer, R. E., Complement alterations in inflammatory bowel disease, *Gastroenterology*, 76, 1374, 1979.
323. Ward, M. and Eastwood, M. A., Serum complement components C3 and C4 in inflammatory bowel disease, *Gut*, 15, 835, 1974.
324. Potter, B. J., Mee, A. S., Hodgson, H. J. F., and Jewell, D. P., Clq metabolism in patients with inflammatory bowel disease, *Gut*, 19, 443, 1978.
325. Teisberg, P. and Gjone, E., Humoral immune system activity in inflammatory bowel disease, *Scand. J. Gastroenterol.*, 10, 545, 1975.
326. Strickland, R. G., Husby, G., Black, W. C., and Williams, R. C., Peripheral blood and intestinal lymphocyte subpopulations in Crohn's disease, *Gut*, 16, 847, 1975.
327. Ryan, F. P., Smart, R. C., Hodsworth, C. D., and Preston, F. E., Hyposplenism in inflammatory bowel disease, *Gut*, 19, 50, 1978.
328. Binder, H. J., Spiro, H. M., and Thayer, W. R., Delayed hypersensitivity in regional enteritis and ulcerative colitis, *Am. J. Dig. Dis.*, 11, 572, 1966.
329. Meyers, S., Sachar, D. B., Taub, R. N., and Janowitz, H. D., Anergy to dinitrochlorobenzene and depression of T lymphocytes in Crohn's disease and ulcerative colitis, *Gut*, 17, 911, 1976.
330. Aas, J., Huizenga, K. A., Newcomer, A. D., and Shorter, R. G., Inflammatory bowel disease: lymphocyte responses to non-specific stimulation in-vitro, *Scand. J. Gastroenterol.*, 7, 299, 1972.
331. Asquith, P., Kraft, S. C., and Ruthberg, R. M., Lymphocyte responses to non-specific mitogens in inflammatory bowel disease, *Gastroenterology*, 65, I, 1973.
332. Bolton, P. M., James, S. L., Newcombe, R. B., Whitehead, R. H., and Hughes, L. E., The immune competence of patients with inflammatory bowel disease, *Gut*, 15, 213, 1974.
333. Soloft, J., Binder, V., and Gudmand-Hoyer, E., Intestinal immunoglobulins in ulcerative colitis, *Scand. J. Gastroenterol.*, 8, 293, 1983.
334. Heatley, R. V., Rhodes, J., Calcraft, B. J., Whithead, R. H., Field, R., and Newcome, R. G., Immunoglobulin E in rectal mucosa of patients with proctitis, *Lancet*, ii, 1010, 1975.
335. Rhodes, J. M. and Jewell, D. P., Motility of neutrophils and monocytes in Crohn's disease and ulcerative colitis, *Gut*, 24, 73, 1983.
336. Wandall, J. H. and Binder, V., Leucocyte function in ulcerative colitis, *Gut*, 23, 758, 1982.
337. Broberger, O. and Perlmann, P., Autoantibodies in human ulcerative colitis, *J. Exp. Med.*, 110, 657, 1959.
338. Wright, R. S. and Truelove, S. C., Autoimmune reactions in ulcerative colitis, *Gut*, 7, 32, 1966.
339. Broberger, O. and Perlmann, P., In-vitro studies of ulcerative colitis. I. Reaction of patients serum with human foetal colon cells in tissue culture, *J. Exp. Med.*, 117, 705, 1963.
340. Lagercrantz, R., Hammarstrom, S., Perlmann, P., and Gustafsson, B. E., Immunological studies in ulcerative colitis. IV. Origin of autoantibodies, *J. Exp. Med.*, 128, 1339, 1968.
341. Perlmann, P., Hammarstrom, S., Lagercrantz, R., and Campbell, D., Autoantibodies to colon in rats and human ulcerative colitis: Cross-reactivity with *Escherichia coli* 014 antigen, *Proc. Soc. Exp. Biol. (NY)*, 125, 975, 1967.
342. McGiven, A. R. T., Ghose, T., and Nairn, R. C., Autoantibodies in ulcerative colitis, *Br. Med. J.*, 2, 19, 1967.
343. Monteiro, E., Fossey, J., Shiner, M., Drasar, B. S., and Allison, A. C., Antibacterial antibodies in rectal and colonic mucosa in ulcerative colitis, *Lancet*, 1, 249, 1971.
344. Hunt, P. S. and Trotter, S., Lymphoblastic response to autologous colon epithelial cells in ulcerative colitis *in-vitro*, *Gut*, 14, 875, 1973.
345. Eckhardt, R., Heinisch, M., and Meyer-Zum-Buschenfelde, K. H., Cellular immune reactions against common antigens, small intestine, and colon antigen in patients with Crohn's disease, ulcerative colitis and cirrhosis of the liver, *Scand. J. Gastroenterol.*, 11, 49, 1976.
346. Stefani, S. and Fink, S., Effects of *E. coli* antigens, tuberculin and phytohaemagglutinin upon ulcerative colitis lymphocytes, *Gut*, 8, 249, 1967.
347. Cooke, E. M., Ewins, S. P., Hiwel-Jones, J., and Lennard-Jones, J. E., Properties of strains of *E. coli* carried in different phases of ulcerative colitis, *Gut*, 15, 143, 1974.

348. Pinder, I. F., Lee, R. J., Dixon, M. F., Cooke, E. M., and Azon, A. T. R., Adhesion of *E. coli* to cultured colonoscopic biopsies from patients with ulcerative colitis, *Gut,* 24, 10, 1983.
349. Cave, D. R., Mitchell, D. N., and Brooke, B. N., Evidence of an agent transmissible from ulcerative colitis tissue, *Lancet,* 1, 1311, 1976.
350. Gitnick, G. L., Rosen, V. J., Arthur, M. H., and Hertweck, S. A., Evidence for the isolation of a new virus from ulcerative colitis patients. Comparison with virus derived from Crohn's disease, *Dig. Dis. Sci.,* 24, 609, 1979.
351. Morain, C. O., Prestage, H., Harrison, P., Levi, A. J., and Tyrrell, D. A. J., Cytopathic effects in cultures innoculated with material from Crohn's disease, *Gut,* 22, 823, 1981.
352. Roche, J. K. and Huang, E. S., Viral DNA in inflammatory bowel disease. CMV-Bearing cells as a target for immune-mediated enterocytolysis, *Gastroenterology,* 72, 228, 1977.
353. Roche, J. K., Wold, W. S. M., Sanders, P. R., Mackey, J. K., and Green, M., Chronic inflammatory bowel disease: absence of adenovirus DNA as established by molecular hybridization, *Gastroenterology,* 81, 853, 1981.
354. Wright, R., and Truelove, S. C., A controlled therapeutic trial of various diets in ulcerative colitis, *Br. Med. J.,* 2, 138, 1965.
355. Wright, R. and Truelove, S. C., Circulating antibodies to dietary proteins in ulcerative colitis., *Br. Med. J.,* 2, 142, 1965.
356. Jewell, D. P. and Truelove, S. C., Circulating antibodies to cows milk proteins in ulcerative colitis, *Gut,* 13, 796, 1972.
357. Brignola, C., Miniero, R., Campieri, M., Bazzocchi, G., Veggetti, S., Fois, F., Farruggia, P., and Lanfranchi, G. A., PRIST and RAST in inflammatory bowel disease, paper presented at 12th Int. Cong. Gastroenterol., Lisbon, September 1984, 531.
358. Harries, A. D., Baird, A., and Rhodes, J., Non-smoking: a feature of ulcerative colitis, *Br. Med. J.,* 284, 706, 1982.
359. Logan, R. F. A., Edmond, M., Somerville, K. W., and Langman, M. J. S., Smoking and ulcerative colitis, *Br. Med. J.,* 288, 751, 1984.
360. Chesner, I., Williams, A., Osman, J., and Asquith, P., Pulmonary function in patients with ulcerative colitis, paper presented at 12th Int. Congr. Gastroenterol., Lisbon, September 1984, 964.

Chapter 6

DIAGNOSIS OF FOOD INTOLERANCE AND ALLERGY

Maurice H. Lessof

TABLE OF CONTENTS

I. Introduction 70
A. Clinical Patterns 70

II. Diagnosis in Childhood 70
A. Inborn Errors of Digestion 70
1. Disorders of Amino Acid and Intermediary Metabolism 71
B. Gastrointestinal Reactions 72
C. Skin Reactions 73
D. Asthma and Rhinitis 74
E. Migraine and Epilepsy 74
F. Hyperactivity 75

III. Diagnosis in Adults 75
A. Syndromes in Adult Life 75
1. Potentiating Factors 77
a. Food Toxicity in Predisposed Subjects 77
2. Pharmacological Effects 78
3. Other Reactions 78
B. Changes with the Storage and Processing of Food 78

IV. Methods of Diagnosis 79
A. Place of Diet in Diagnosis 79
B. Unorthodox and Negative Tests 80

References 81

I. INTRODUCTION

The joint report of the Royal College of Physicians and the British Nutrition Foundation[1] defined food intolerance as a reproducible, unpleasant (i.e., adverse) reaction to a specific food or food ingredient which is not psychologically based. Unlike phychological symptoms, food intolerant reactions occur even when the food is given in an unrecognized form e.g., when it is disguised by flavoring and given as a purée. "Food allergy" is defined as a form of food intolerance in which there is also evidence of an abnormal immunological reaction to the food. "Food aversion" is either an avoidance of food for psychological reasons or can include psychologically induced symptoms in which an unpleasant bodily reaction is caused by emotional mechanisms rather than by the food itself.

Food intolerance which is reproducible on more than one occasion may nevertheless arise in several different ways — as a result of enzyme defects, pharmacological causes, the effects of irritants or toxins (especially when the mucosa is diseased), or the fermentation of unabsorbed food residues in the lower bowel. Allergy or the presence of other immunological abnormalities can be demonstrated only in a minority of cases, most commonly in association with other evidence of allergic disease. Confirmatory evidence of allergy is provided by the detection of immunoglobulin E (IgE) antibodies which react with the appropriate food, but laboratory test methods are less satisfactory for most of the other mechanisms of food intolerance.

It remains to be established whether the relative infrequency with which an immunological reaction can be demonstrated is due to the inadequancy of test methods or whether immunological causes are uncommon. In gluten enteropathy, where the relationship to a specific food is proven, diagnostic confirmation is more readily obtained from a histological method (i.e., biopsy evidence of jejunal mucosal atrophy) than from evidence of antibody formation — although antibodies to gluten fractions or to reticulin are indeed a feature of the disease.

A. Clinical Patterns

The most easily diagnosed food intolerant reactions are those which occur within a few minutes, and the cause and effect are often most easily established in childhood (see Table 1). Reactions which occur within an hour include vomiting and other gastrointestinal reactions as well as anaphylactic collapse, angioedema, urticaria, or asthma. In children, symptoms which accompany food allergy include limb pains and migraine; despite their nonspecific nature, epilepsy, enuresis, irritability, and hyperactivity have been claimed to be significant association.[2,3] In the adult, early reactions tend to be described in more detail and include swelling of the lips, tingling of the mouth or throat, vomiting and abdominal pain, and complaints of abdominal bloating, constipation, diarrhea, or the development of fatty stools. It has also been claimed that food may provoke pains in the joints or exacerbate the symptoms of rheumatoid arthritis.[4,5]

II. DIAGNOSIS IN CHILDHOOD

A. Inborn Errors of Digestion

Inborn errors of digestion or absorption can affect the metabolism of carbohydrate, fat, or protein.[6] The most frequent symptom is watery diarrhea, and it may be difficult to distinguish between enzyme deficiencies and other causes of food intolerance. Profuse diarrhea in the neonatal period may suggest severe congenital disorders such as glucose-galactose malabsorption, but the symptoms vary considerably in severity and can present when there is a slow decline in enzyme activity later in childhood, as in the

Table 1
PROVEN AND UNPROVEN REACTIONS TO FOOD IN CHILDHOOD

Timing of the reaction to food	Reaction patterns	Proof that relationship exists
Immediate	Anaphylaxis Angioedema Urticaria	Relationship obvious except when due to azo dyes and preservatives
Immediate and/or late	Vomiting/diarrhea Failure to thrive Eczema Rhinitis Asthma	Difficult — often established only by controlled challenge
Not established	Infantile colic Migraine ± epilepsy	Variable association with food intolerance
	Hyperactivity Essential reactive hypoglycemia	No established association with food intolerance
Nonexistent	Food intolerance by proxy	Requires careful assessment by psychiatrist and physician

Data based on Joint Committee Report, *J. R. Coll. Physicians*, 18, 83, 1984.

acquired type of hypolactasia. Withdrawal of the offending sugar leads to an improvement of symptoms, and a diagnosis can be established by giving a challenge with the appropriate material, observing the clinical response, and measuring stool sugars or breath hydrogen. Small intestinal biopsy samples can be used for measurements of lactase activity or the presence of sucrase-isomaltase.

The enzyme defects which have so far been mentioned give rise to symptoms because of the secondary effects of unabsorbed food residues. Symptoms can also arise because of a lack of essential nutrients or because of an accumulation of toxic intermediate products which cannot be processed through the normal metabolic pathways.[7]

In the inherited disorders of protein digestion, a deficiency of such enzymes as enterokinase and trypsinogen can lead to a failure to thrive, the production of offensive stools, hypoproteinemia and anemia.[8] Deficiencies of amino acid absorption can also lead to protein intolerance,[9] but a number of neuropsychiatric and other symptoms could result from the absorption of breakdown products from unabsorbed amino acids.[10] Similar mechanisms may operate where there is a malabsorption of fat, whether due to a deficiency of such enzymes as lipase and cholelipase or due to pancreatic disease.[11]

Despite the rarity of most inborn errors of metabolism, a few are sufficiently common to be important causes of nonspecific symptoms of food intolerance, especially among non-Caucasian people. Hemolytic anemia due to glucose-6-phosphate dehydrogenase deficiency is seen in 1% or more of certain ethnic populations, but this is much less common than adult-onset lactase deficiency, which has a prevalence of up to 90% in some communities. Intolerance to alcohol due to aldehyde dehydrogenase deficiency is seen in 40% or more of some Asian communities.[12]

1. Disorders of Amino Acid and Intermediary Metabolism

Rarely do enzyme defects which prevent the normal metabolism of amino acids lead to toxic levels of ammonia in the blood or cause an accumulation of organic acids. The effects are mainly seen in the central nervous system and may lead to a toxic encephalopathy which is potentially fatal. Those with less severe disease can still present in the first year of life because of loss of appetite, vomiting, delayed development, and later, ataxia and slurring of speech. Symptoms can be exacerbated by protein, and mothers who become aware of this select a low-protein diet without necessarily being advised to do so.

B. Gastrointestinal Reactions

The association between metabolic disorders and allergic disease may be clearly demonstrable in the presence of an associated asthma and rhinitis, eczema, or other immediate reactions such as urticaria or angioedema; though even here it may be difficult to exclude pharmacological effects (e.g., to aspirin) which closely mimic allergic disease.[13] In those conditions in which vomiting and gastrointestinal symptoms occur in isolation, diagnosis may be more difficult.

In the infant, a distinction between normal and abnormal bowel function can be difficult to judge. Almost all babies regurgitate some milk which may be regarded as a normal variant, providing it does not interfere with nutrition. Food intolerance is merely one of a number of causes of severe vomiting and a failure to thrive, but where there is an average weight gain of less than 150 g/week in the first 3 months of life, further investigation is required. Crying attacks with legs drawn up and a red face suggest abdominal colic which can draw attention to other eivdence of a gastrointestinal disturbance, but the dividing line between the normal and the abnormal is often misunderstood. This is particularly so in the case of diarrhea in babies, since breast-fed babies commonly have up to 10 to 12 stools daily and may have explosive stools with mucus in the first few weeks of life. In the bottle-fed baby, a sudden change to a diarrhea stool can be more obvious and is likely to be due to infection. Gastrointestinal reactions to cow's milk or later to other foods may therefore deserve consideration only after these more common problems have been excluded. Nevertheless, there may occasionally be some very characteristic features such as blood in the stools in association with a milk-induced colitis, a condition which differs from ulcerative colitis and responds to milk withdrawal.[14,15]

Of those children who have food intolerance, only a minority have gastrointestinal symptoms,[16] but those who do often have or subsequently develop other more obvious atopic disorders. Nevertheless, skin tests, total IgE, and IgG antibody measurements are of poor diagnostic value.[16,17] A small intestinal biopsy can occasionally provide evidence of mucosal damage in cow's milk protein intolerance[17] or in relationship to soya, chicken, rice, fish, or egg intolerance,[18,19] but in other cases it may be necessary to establish the diagnosis of food intolerance by resorting to dietary exclusion followed by rechallenge along the lines recommended by Goldman and colleagues.[20]

Celiac disease results from an intolerance of the gluten proteins in wheat, oats, rye, or barley which is usually lifelong and most commonly presents before the age of 2 years with abnormal stools, anorexia, vomiting, and abdominal distension or with such symptoms as irritability and muscle wasting. The condition can present at any age, however, and symptoms include constipation, episodes of diarrhea, iron-deficiency anemia, rickets, and short stature. In this case, evidence of small intestinal mucosal damage on biopsy is a requirement before the diagnosis can be confirmed. It is of interest that the small intestine enteropathy which is seen in celiac disease is histologically very similar to other types of food-induced small intestine enteropathy, but the clinical features show some striking differences. In addition to those mentioned, it is sometimes associated with the characteristic skin rash of "dermatitis herpetiformis" but not with eczema or other allergic features.

Table 2
CAUSES OF URTICARIA

Cause	Nature of reaction
Allergic	IgE-mediated mast cell activation
Pharmacological	Response to salicylate, food amines, etc.
Complement enzyme activation	Immune complex deposition and intrinsic defects of complement system.
Pseudoallergic mediator release	Physical and cholinergic urticaria, provoked by cold, heat, pressure, stress, etc.

C. Skin Reactions

Skin rashes are a common feature of infancy and childhood, often as a nonspecific reaction to injury or infection. The "nappy rash" which affects most babies sooner or later consists of perineal soreness and rash which is usually due to ammonia dermatitis, *Candida* infection, or seborrheic dermatitis. Atopic dermatitis, giving the classical appearance of eczema, is also relatively common and affects 5% of children but rarely before 6 weeks of age. Maculopapular rashes of less specific nature occur commonly through childhood, especially after viral infections, when they are often mistakenly attributed to antibiotic allergy. Transient urticaria is also remarkably common and can have a number of causes (see Table 2). Not uncommonly it is postinfective, and reactions to β-hemolytic streptocococci, *Campylobacter,*[21] or other infective agents may lead to inappropriate investigation for food allergy.

Urticaria, angioedema, or, in the most severe cases, an anaphylactic reaction may occur so immediately after taking an offending food that diagnosis can be simple and further tests superfluous. Nevertheless, skin prick tests are usually positive, and IgE antibodies may be detectable by such methods as the radioallergosorbent test or enzyme-linked immunosorbent assay. The foods most commonly involved include eggs, various nuts, and fish. In the most severe cases, food challenge can provoke so severe a reaction that it is to be avoided.

At one time or another, more than 20% of the population have urticaria or angioedema. These self-limited urticarial episodes are common in childhood, but chronic recurring skin reactions may sometimes persist for 3 months or more. In most children (but not in adults) the causes are identifiable and incude foods, drugs, inhalant allergens, physical agents (e.g., heat and cold), emotional stress, and, exceptionally, an hereditary deficiency of C1 esterase inhibitor. Other types of inherited defects may also be detectable in atopic patients, including an opsonizing defect which interferes with the phagocytic function of leukocytes[22] and a deficiency of the second component of complement.[23]

As far as urticaria is concerned, specific foods have often been implicated. Food additives such as tartrazine, sunset yellow, and benzoic acid are so regularly ingested by children that their relationship to recurring urticaria may not at first be obvious. When no other cause of chronic urticaria can be found, it is useful to try a diet which is free of azo dyes and preservatives and can lead to remission in something like 50% of cases.[24] Of those patients who lose their symptoms while on a diet, less than half react to coloring matter or benzoate when a double-blind challenge is arranged. While this may not necessarily exclude the possibility that food additives were responsible for maintaining a child's urticaria, most children who fail to react on challenge can be reestablished on a normal diet without a relapse of symptoms.

Eczema provides a much more insidious form of rash which, although complex in its origin, is increasingly found to be associated with food intolerance or allergy.[25] Although the purely breast-fed child can develop eczema — sometimes in response to food proteins absorbed through the mother's milk — early weaning has been claimed to play a part. If other forms of treatment are unsuccessful, dietary "exclusion" measures, though tedious, can sometimes be effective both in diagnosis and treatment.

Positive skin tests to foods have been claimed to provide a useful screening test in children with atopic dermatitis and high IgE levels and have been used in the selection of suspect foods to be eliminated from the diet for 10 to 14 days.[26] On rechallenge, a positive reaction has been reported in more than half of the children tested, as indicated by pruritis and macular or maculopapular rash involving 5% or more of the body surface. This pruritis and erythema led to scratching, and eczematous lesions were noted to develop subsequently.

The only controlled trial of dietary treatment in eczema showed a clear advantage for children treated with a diet which excluded egg, cow's milk, chicken, and beef.[27] A dramatic improvement has also been reported in five out of ten children with very severe eczema treated with elemental diets.[28] Diets are, however, difficult to maintain even when the parents are highly motivated.[29]

D. Asthma and Rhinitis

The mucosa of the respiratory tract is more likely to respond to inhaled allergens than to foods. Nevertheless, it is by no means uncommon for patients to complain of sneezing reactions after food or for patients with allergic asthma to report that foods are among the agents which can provoke asthmatic attacks. While the smell of the relevant food appears to provoke the reaction in many cases, a gastrointestinal challenge has also been shown to be capable of causing rhinitis in double-blind studies in which milk was introduced into the stomach through a nasogastric tube.[30]

In suspected cases of respiratory allergy due to food the use of elimination diets and rechallenge methods can be cumbersome. Furthermore, pharmacological approaches to therapy are relatively simple and efficacious regardless of the specific provoking causes. Diagnostic challenge tests may not therefore be worth undertaking except in difficult cases unless there is a strong suspicion that specific foods are among the factors which provoke an asthmatic attack. Unfortunately, even where the history is clear, challenge tests within a hospital setting may fail to provide convincing evidence, and the response may appear to be below the threshold of clinical detection. It has been noted, however, that challenge tests with food which may not produce a change in lung function can nevertheless increase bronchial reactivity to small amounts of inhaled histamine.[31]

E. Migraine and Epilepsy

The relationship between food and migraine has been known for more than a century. While the foods which are responsible include cheeses with a very high content of vasoactive amines, it has also been claimed that allergy may be involved.[32] In a report of a double-blind placebo-controlled trial,[33] it has been shown that children with severe migraine may have their attacks provoked by foods which are not known to contain amines and are unlikely to have a pharmacological effect but are, on the other hand, well known to be capable of causing allergic reactions. Although laboratory and skin tests were negative in this trial, the children studied and members of their families had a high prevalence of atopy and atopic diseases. A strong case has therefore been made for prescribing an elimination diet in children with severe migraine so that if the migraine attacks cease, this can provide the basis for rechallenge with a succession of foods in order to identify those which are capable of triggering migraine in an individual case. An incidental finding of this study was that children successfully treated by diet showed an improvement in other symptoms such as abdominal pain and eczema and that in the occasional case in which there were associated fits or hyperkinetic behavior, this also improved. Furthermore, those who were successfully treated by diet no longer developed migraine when excited or when exposed to noise, bright lights, or other nonspecific stimuli which had previously caused attacks.

F. Hyperactivity

There has been much controversy over the question of whether hyperactive children who exhibit disruptive behavior may on occasion be suffering from food intolerance. An incidence as high as 25% has been claimed in some schools,[34] and even the lower estimate of 3 to 10% in schools in the U.S.[35] is still much higher than that in the U.K. This suggests that psychosocial or other factors may account for the great variation in the incidence in school communities regardless of differences in diet which, in general, are not known to differ greatly between different centers in the U.S. and in the U.K. (see Chapter 7 for further details).

The use of a diet free of additives and salicylates has been extensively encouraged as a means of diagnosing hyperactivity due to food intolerance, but although mood alteration may accompany the more distressing reactions to foods such as migraine, urticaria, eczema, and diarrhea,[33] the suggestion that mood alteration can be the sole expression of food intolerance remains controversial. A recent study of 17 healthy children presenting at an allergy clinic showed that the diets of children can be severely restricted by mothers who mistakenly believe that food allergy is the cause of a wide range of unsubstantiated symptoms.[36] In many cases, the mother's belief is reinforced by organizations which claim to have special techniques for the diagnosis of food intolerance, whereas a clinical assessment has suggested that these may be cases of "food intolerance by proxy."[37]

III. DIAGNOSIS IN ADULTS

A. Syndromes in Adult Life

By the time adult life is reached, sensitization may sometimes be present to a very wide range of ingested substances. This is reflected in the very large number of foods which have not been reported as being capable of provoking specific adverse reactions in sensitive individuals. An abbreviated list of these foods has been provided in Table 3.

Gastrointestinal symptoms are common in adults who have an "irritable bowel syndrome" after ingesting certain foods, but these symptoms are not necessarily provoked by the same foods as in childhood, the most common being wheat (in patients with a normal jejunal biopsy), corn, dairy products, coffee, tea, and citrus fruits. By way of contrast, patients who react to egg, nuts, or fish often develop asthma, eczema, angioedema, or urticaria, suggesting that these foods provoke an allergic response. This is further supported by their association with positive skin or radioallergosorbent tests in over 70% of cases.[38] Milk and dairy products, while they may provoke similar reactions, have been reported as giving positive skin or radioallergosorbent tests only in about 30% of cases. While some form of delayed immunological reaction may account for cases with negative allergy tests, it is also possible that reactions are occurring — as in the irritable bowel syndrome — which are not due to immunological causes of any kind. Both immunological and nonimmunological mechanisms could also explain

Table 3
FOOD ALLERGY AND INTOLERANCE

Foods Commonly Involved

Cow's milk	Wheat/cereals/flour/yeast	Coffee/tea
Hen's egg	Chocolate	Preservatives
Fish/shellfish	Pork/bacon/tenderized meat	Artificial colors

Other Foods Reported as Causing Reactions

Aniseed	Clove	Pea
Apple	Fennel	Peach
Artichoke	Filbert	Peppers (various)
Banana	Garlic	Potato
Beans (various)	Ginger	Seeds (caraway, dill, poppy, sunflower)
Beet	Herbs (bay, sage, thyme)	Sesame
Berries (various)	Honey	Soya
Celery	Horseradish	Sweet potato
Camomile	Hops	Tapioca
Chestnut	Mango	Vanilla
Chicken	Millet	
Chicory	Mustard	
Cinnamon	Nutmeg	

Data from Joint Committee Report, *J. R. Coll. Physicians*, 18, 83, 1984.

the variety of reactions which are seen to wheat and yeast products, soya, and chocolate.[39] Nonimmunological causes of food intolerance due to enzyme deficiencies or pharmacological effects have already been mentioned but fail to account for all the food-induced symptoms which have been described. For example, a relative intolerance to substantial amounts of fatty food has been described in otherwise healthy subjects.[40]

In the case of some of the less common syndromes of adult life, the ability of a food to provoke exacerbations of the disease can only be established by trial and error. Tests for IgE antibodies can help to establish the presence of an immunological component, but in the case of eosinophilic gastroenteritis[41] or rectal bleeding in the case of patients with hemorrhagic proctitis,[42] evidence of a classical allergic response may be lacking. From the point of view of diagnosis, the exacerbating role of specific foods can sometimes be demonstrated in such cases, and the same may be true of patients with the nephrotic syndrome who have been reported to develop relapses on drinking milk[43] or of patients in whom a low blood platelet count can be reversed on a milk-free diet.[44]

The differences between reactions in childhood and in adult life are seen in virtually every organ system which is affected, and once again it may be that the symptoms of intolerance are due to a number of different mechanisms. For example, patients with gastrointestinal symptoms which were thought to be related to specific foods were in one study challenged with capsules containing either the suspect food or placebo.[45] Only 3 out of 19 patients reacted to the food, and these were patients who had other IgE-mediated reactions. In another study, patients with nausea, bloating, abdominal pain, and either constipation or diarrhea were investigated in order to exclude alactasia or gastrointestinal disease and then challenged with flavored purée preparations in a double-blind study.[46] As many as two thirds developed gastrointestinal symptoms after specific foods, sometimes accompanied by objective evidence of an increased rectal release of prostaglandins. The differences between one study and another are difficult to explain, but it is possible that small encapsulated quantities of food are sufficient to trigger a reaction in patients with food allergy, whereas in other types of food intolerance it may be preferable to rely on larger quantities or the repeated administration of the appropriate food or foods. Since some of the symptoms depend on the release of intestinal gas as a result of the bacterial fermentation of unabsorbed food residues,[47] symptoms due to this cause may appear only after an interval of some hours. Colonic bacteria can both produce and consume hydrogen,[48] and changes in bacterial flora due to infection or the use of antibiotics might therefore be suspected in patients who date the onset of their symptoms to a gastrointestinal infection.

1. Potentiating Factors

The complex nature of food reactions has been noted both in children and adults. Even in well-documented anaphylactic reactions to shellfish in a patient with demonstrable IgE antibodies, it has been shown that an anaphylactic response may occur only when the meal is followed by exercise.[49] A similar relationship to exercise has also been described in three patients whose allergy to celery led to symptoms only after exercise was taken.[50]

Food-induced migraine, whether provoked by allergy or by a pharmacological response to tyramine and other amines,[51] is most likely to develop in a few well-defined circumstances which do not depend on the food alone. The most common precipitating factor is stress, but lack of food can also precipitate migraine in those who are predisposed.[52] It has also been noted that an attack of migraine may be followed by a refractory period, after which prodromal symptoms begin to recur, signaling a susceptibility to further migraine episodes.[53] Some patients become irritable or depressed, while others feel elated, sleepy, or hungry. Cravings for sweet or carbohydrate food may be noted the day or the evening before an attack is due.[53]

The tendency for joint pains to develop after food intake in predisposed subjects is also the result of complex factors. In the disturbed uric acid metabolism of gout, alcohol can both increase the synthesis of urate[54] and reduce its urinary excretion.[55] In the case of gout, the effect of alcohol thus appears to have a metabolic basis, but not all joint pains which follow food intake can be similarly explained. It has been suggested that an exacerbation of seronegative rheumatoid arthritis after milk may be related to an impaired ability to metabolize immune complexes,[5] and it is possible that food containing immune complexes can activate platelets and cause a release of serotonin.[4] As yet, however, there is insufficient evidence to justify the use of immune complex tests or serotonin measurements for diagnostic purposes.

a. Food Toxicity in Predisposed Subjects

Occasional examples have been noted in which foods or food additives can be selectively toxic to a few individuals. This is reminiscent of the variable response to drugs which occurs in individuals characterized as "slow acetylators", in whom variations in enzyme activity may account for an increased susceptibility to drug effects. It now appears that variations in enzyme activity can in a somewhat similar way predispose to the adverse effects which occur after specific foods. Measurements of glucose-6-phosphate dehydrogenase levels may thus identify subjects who are likely to develop hemolytic anemia after eating fava beans or who develop anemia and abnormal liver function after eating foods which have been colored with the dye orange-RN.[56] It has also been suggested that individuals may vary in their susceptibility to the cholinesterase-inhibiting effect of food which has been sprayed with insecticides,[57] and the possibility of identifying susceptible subjects by means of other enzyme measurements remains to be explored. In most cases, however, an individual's susceptibility to reactions associated with foods remains unexplained. The effect of challenge tests remains the basis on which food intolerance can be confirmed, and this remains so whether the effects are pharmacological or due to enzyme defects, allergy, or some other abnormality.

2. Pharmacological Effects

The importance of pharmacological effects have probably been underestimated in the past. Caffeine, the most popular and widely used stimulant drug in the world, has its pharmacological effects at a dose of about 200 mg, which may be contained in perhaps three cups of tea or two of reasonably strong coffee. In toxic doses it can induce extrasystoles or paroxysmal tachycardia,[58] tremor, sweating, headache, and tachypnea.[59] Tea or coffee can also provoke esophageal reflux, nausea, vomiting, or diarrhea in a few subjects,[60] and restless or "jittery" legs have also been attributed to caffeine effects.[61] As severe withdrawal symptoms can occur, the caffeine intake should be tailed off and stopped, and then, after an interval, a further challenge should be given in full doses.

Pharmacological effects may also be apparent after the ingestion of foods which contain vasoactive amines. High concentrations of tyramine (1 to 2 mg/g) are present in some cheeses and pickled fish. Phenylethylamine is found in chocolate, and citrus fruit contains octopamine and synephrine. It has been suggested that, in susceptible subjects, through their effects on blood vessels and indirectly by the liberation of adrenaline and noradrenaline from nerve endings, these substances can cause facial flushing and urticaria or can precipitate headaches. In a controlled study in which either tyramine or lactose tablets were given to migraine sufferers, headache was provoked in 80 out of 100 subjects who received 125 mg of tyramine, whereas lactose tablets produced headache in only 6 out of 66.[51]

3. Other Reactions

Nonimmunological, "pseudoallergic" reactions are being recognized in increasing numbers. There has been much discussion on the ability of absorbed food products either to sustain histamine or other amine activity in the body or to provoke the release of histamine and other mediators. Since histamine cannot readily penetrate the mucosal barrier and high levels in the portal venous blood may not reach the systemic circulation,[62] it is possible that such effects are only able to occur if the amount ingested is high or if there is some failure of function in the gut mucosa or the liver. Regardless of these considerations and the fact that the same conditions may not be reproducible from day to day, a firm diagnosis can only depend on the clinical response to an appropriate food challenge or on obtaining evidence of mediator release or some other indication of a subclinical response. A good example of this is seen in those children who develop an increased bronchial reactivity to histamine after taking cola drinks to which they are sensitive.[31] The same principle applies to reactions caused by monosodium glutamate[63,64] or other food additives.

B. Changes with the Storage and Processing of Food

In choosing the form in which foods are to be given for challenge purposes, it may be important to recognize the changes which can be brought about by storage and processing. Bleumink[65] reported intolerance to ripe (but not green) tomtoes, which was later shown to be caused by a glycoprotein produced in the tomato skin by a nonenzymatic (Maillard) browning reaction.[66] Others have noted that decomposed foods, e.g., rancid fats, may be a cause of urticaria.[67] Although histamine does not normally reach the circulation in appreciable quantities, old fermented foods including cheeses and badly stored scombroid fish such as mackerel are capable of producing unpleasant reactions which have been well documented.[68-70] Diagnosis may in this case depend on the history because it may not be practical to attempt to reproduce the symptoms on rechallenge. Clinically, the symptoms cannot be distinguished from an allergic manifestation and in the case of scombroid poisoning can include urticaria, nausea, vomiting, facial flushing, intense headache, epigastric pain, a burning sensation in the throat, dysphagia, thirst, and lip swelling. The incubation period for a reaction varies from 10 min to 2 hr.[71] and as the histamine concentration in the scombroid fish may rise to 100 mg/100 g if it is not stored in the cold, histamine poisoning has been blamed. However, since nonscombroid fish sometimes contain high concentrations of histamine but do not cause this type of poisoning, histamine cannot be the only substance involved in the reaction.[72]

It is not only histamine which is suspect but also tyramine, which is present in cheese, chocolate, liver, sausages, broad beans, and pickled herrings. All of these foods have been thought to have pharmacological effects on occasions, especially in patients receiving monoamine oxidase-inhibiting drugs. The capacity to provoke reactions may, however, be modified by the type of processing to which certain foods — for example, beans and legumes — have been subjected. Kidney beans contain variable amounts of protein (lectins) which have the ability to agglutinate RBC and are toxic in other ways; since lectins are heat labile, cooking will eliminate their toxic properties.[73] Heat also appears to inactivate chlorogenic acid in oranges and coffee[74] and also components of potato which are capable of causing skin reactions.[75] Solvent dehydration of bananas has a similar inactivating effect.[76]

Attempts to arrange diagnostic tests may therefore depend not only on identifying the appropriate food for challenge purposes but on providing it in the form in which a reaction can best be provoked. This does not apply equally to all substances. Many of the food "allergens" are relatively stable glycoproteins. Skin-reactive components in egg, tomatoes, and various fish appear to be thermostable,[66] as are some of the proteins in peas, beans, and peanuts.[77]

IV. METHODS OF DIAGNOSIS

A. Place of Diet in Diagnosis

Diagnostic diets tend to be time consuming and difficult. They are not therefore indicated where the symptoms are mild and controllable by simple measures or when the symptoms of intolerance are known to be provoked by a single, avoidable food. Analysis of the dietary history may be supplemented by a food diary — a record of food and drink taken over a period of days — and if the opportunity arises, the elimination of one or two suspect foods may be attempted, followed by rechallenge if the symptoms are successfully eliminated. Otherwise, a more general elimination diet can be chosen, using either an extremely restricted diet of lamb, pears, rice, and water[45] or eliminating those foods which are most commonly associated with adverse reactions, such as milk products, eggs, fish, pork, wheat products, nuts, coffee, tea, chocolate, alcohol, and artificially colored or preserved foods. Only if the symptoms disappear within a period of 1 to 3 weeks is the possibility of food intolerance worth pursuing through the stepwise reintroduction, at intervals of a few days, of substantial and repeated quantities of each of the eliminated foods.

The choice of foods which can be used in an elimination diet is necessarily arbitrary. Since a somewhat different range of foods have been identified as provoking the irritable bowel syndrome, Hunter and colleagues[46] use an elimination diet which excludes wheat, potato, dairy products, citrus fruits, and coffee but does not exclude meat or fish. In the investigation of childhood migraine, Egger et al.[33] have suggested a diet which allows one meat (lamb or chicken), one carbohydrate food (rice or potato), one fruit (banana or apple), one vegetable (brassica), water, and vitamin supplements.

Those who show no improvement after 3 or 4 weeks are offered a second diet which has no foods in common with the first.

If there is no response, despite strict adherence to the diet, the diagnosis of food intolerance can usually be excluded. Exceptionally, an elemental diet may be needed, but few patients are able to tolerate this for long. Since their use reduces the bulk of intestinal secretions, they may dramatically reduce the symptoms associated with such factors as intestinal obstruction, and this should be borne in mind when the results come to be analyzed.

When the results of dietary elimination and challenge have led to a provisional diagnosis of food intolerance, the reintroduction of foods should first be carried out openly and then for confirmatory purposes in disguised form so that they are not identifiable by the subject. Where there is a possibility of a psychologically based food aversion, it may not be possible to make a firm diagnosis without double-blind challenge tests in which the patient is given in random sequence the disguised test food or a specially constituted food which is indistinguishable in color, taste, texture, or appearances.[46]

B. Unorthodox and Negative Tests

A number of other test methods have been the subject of extravagant claims but have not been shown to be of value. The pulse test was described by Coca[78] and depends on the interpretation of a rise in pulse rate to indicate foods to which a patient is intolerant. While severe food reactions may indeed be accompanied by a tachycardia, this is also seen in patients who hyperventilate and in numerous other circumstances.

Drops of food solutions administered under the tongue have also been claimed to be capable of eliciting diagnostic evidence of food hypersensitivity. While it is true that a positive, local reaction may be obtained in patients with immediate reactions of the oral urticaria type, such patients react equally well to skin prick tests with the appropriate food extracts.[79] In practice, the response to such tests has failed to discriminate between control materials and food extracts.[80-82]

The skin response to intradermal injections of food extracts has also been used for diagnostic purposes and in the case of a very few foods has given a useful indication of an IgE-mediated reaction. The Rinkel technique uses a much wider range of solutions which are poorly characterized but are nevertheless "titrated" at different concentrations to provide evidence of food allergy. Whereas skin test evidence of IgE-mediated reactions can be useful in patients with the immediate type of reaction, the claims of Rinkel's followers go well beyond this group of patients and have not been validated either for diagnosis or treatment.[83]

It has also been claimed that "cytotoxic" food tests can be carried out for diagnostic purposes and that the WBC of food-allergic patients will die and disintegrate in the presence of the food to which the patient is sensitive.[84] Day-to-day fluctuations in the results of these tests raise questions about their validity,[85] and one British laboratory has failed to obtain reproducible results on duplicate blood samples taken from the same subjects at the same time.[86] While an effect of allergens on WBC may indeed be demonstrable if appropriate methods are developed for the detection of basophil degranulation,[87] "cytotoxic" tests based on Black's method appear to be both outmoded in concept and misleading in practice.

One of the recurring problems of assessing food-intolerant reactions remains the distinction between true food intolerance and food aversion of various types. In many cases, a patient who is apprehensive about the likelihood of a reaction to a specific food can be shown to develop symptoms on hyperventilating in association with respiratory alkalosis. The symptoms range from paresthesia and weakness, to nausea, giddiness, and tachycardia. By asking a patient to hyperventilate for 1 to 2 min, it is possible to assess whether the patient's customary "food allergy" symptoms are reproduced in these circumstances. While it does not follow that the presence of food intolerance and the hyperventilation syndrome are mutually exclusive, the results of a hyperventilation test can be a considerable aid to diagnosis or at least to the need to use blind challenge methods.

REFERENCES

1. Food intolerance and food aversion, Report of Joint Committee of the Royal College of Physicians and British Nutrition Foundation, M. H. Lessof, Chairman, *J. R. Coll. Physicians,* 18, 83, 1984.
2. Minford, A. M. B., Macdonald, A., and Littlewood, J. M., Food intolerance and food allergy in children: a review of 68 cases, *Arch. Dis. Child.,* 57, 742, 1982.
3. Frick, O. L., Controversial concepts and techniques with emphasis on food allergy, in *Allergic Diseases of Infancy, Childhood and Adolescence,* Bierman, C. W. and Pearlman, D. S., Eds., W. B. Saunders, Philadelphia, 1980, 738.
4. Little, C. H., Stewart, A. G., and Fennessy, M. R., Platelet serotonin release in rheumatoid arthritis: a study in food-intolerant patients, *Lancet,* 2, 297, 1983.
5. Parke, A. L. and Hughes, G. R. V., Rheumatoid arthritis and food: a case study, *Br. Med. J.,* 282, 2027, 1981.
6. Harries, J. T., Familial inherited abnormalities, *Clin. Gastroenterol.,* 11, 1, 1982.
7. Stanbury, J. B., Wyngaarden, J. B., Fredrickson, D. S., Goldstein, J. L., and Brown, M. S., Eds., *The Metabolic Basis of Inherited Disease,* 5th ed., McGraw-Hill, New York, 1983.
8. Harries, J. T., Ed., Selective inborn errors of absorption, in *Essentials of Paediatric Gastroenterology,* Churchill Livingstone, Edinburgh, 1977, 199.
9. Walser, M., Urea cycle disorders and other hereditary hyperammonaemic syndromes, in *The Metabolic Basis of Inherited Disease,* 5th ed., Stanbury, J. B., Wyngaarden, J. B., Fredrickson, D. S., Goldstein, J. L., and Brown, M. S., Eds., McGraw-Hill, New York, 1983, 427.
10. Jepson, J., Hartnup disease, in *The Meatbolic Basis of Inherited Disease,* 4th ed., Stanbury, J. B., Wyngaarden, J. B., and Fredrickson, D. S., Eds., McGraw-Hill, New York, 1978, 1563.
11. Muller, D. P. R., Disorders of lipid absorption, *Clin. Gastroenterol.,* 11, 119, 1982.
12. Harada, S., Agarwal, D. P., Goedde, H. W., Tagaki, S., and Ishikawa, B., Possible protective role against alcoholism for aldehyde dehydrogenase isoenzyme deficiency in Japan, *Lancet,* 2, 827, 1982.
13. Asad, S. I., Kemeny, D. M., Youlten, L. J. F., Frankland, A. W., and Lessof, M. H., Effect of aspirin in "aspirin sensitive patients", *Br. Med. J.,* 288, 745, 1984.
14. Gryboski, J. D., Gastrointestinal milk allergy in infants, *Pediatrics,* 40, 354, 1967.
15. Jenkins, H. R., Pincott, J. R., Soothill, J. F., et al., Food allergy: the major cause of infantile colitis, *Arch. Dis. Child.,* 59, 326, 1984.
16. Hill, D. J., Davidson, G. P., Cameron, D. J. S., and Barnes, G. L., The spectrum of cow's milk allergy in childhood, *Acta Paediatr. Scand.,* 68, 847, 1979.
17. Hutchins, P. and Walker-Smith, J. A., The gastrointestinal system, *Clin. Immunol. Allergy,* 2, 43, 1982.
18. Ament, M. E. and Rubin, C. E., Soy protein — another cause of the flat intestinal lesion, *Gastroenterology,* 62, 227, 1972.
19. Vitoria, J. C., Camarero, C., Sojo, A., Ruiz, A., and Rodriguez-Soriano, J., Enteropathy related to fish, rice and chicken, *Arch. Dis. Child.,* 57, 44, 1982.
20. Goldman, A. S., Anderson, D. W., Sellars, W. A., Saperstein, D., Kniker, W. T., and Halpern, S. R., Milk allergy. I. Oral challenge with milk and isolated milk proteins in allergic children, *Pediatrics,* 32, 425, 1963.
21. Bretag, A. H., Archer, R. S., Atkinson, H. M., et al., Circadian urticaria, *Lancet,* 1, 954, 1984.
22. Soothill, J. F. and Harvey, B. A. M., Defective opsonization, a common immunity deficiency, *Arch. Dis. Child.,* 51, 91, 1976.
23. Turner, M. W., Mowbray, J. F., Harvey, B. A. M., Brostoff, J., Wells, R. S., and Soothill, J. F., Defective yeast opsonization and C_2 deficiency in atopic patients, *Clin. Exp. Immunol.,* 34, 253, 1978.
24. Supramanium, G. and Warner, J. O., Abstract from the International Paediatric Association, Manila, 1983.

25. Atherton, D. J., Atopic eczema, *Clin. Immunol. Allergy,* 2, 77, 1982.
26. Sampson, H. A., Role of immediate food hypersensitivity in the pathogenesis of atopic dermatitis, *Allergy Clin. Immunol.,* 71, 473, 1983.
27. Atherton, D. J., Sewell, M., Soothill, J. F., and Wells, R. S., A double-blind controlled crossover trial of an antigen-avoidance diet in atopic eczema, *Lancet,* 1, 401, 1978.
28. Hill, D. J. and Lynch, B. C., Elemental diet in the management of severe eczema in childhood, *Clin. Allergy,* 12, 313, 1982.
29. Anderson, J. A., Non-immunologically-mediated food sensitivity, *Nutr. Rev.,* 42, 109, 1984.
30. Bock, S. A., Lee, W.-Y., Remigio, L. K., and May, C. D., Studies of hypersensitivity reactions to foods in infants and children, *Allergy Clin. Immunol.,* 62, 327, 1978.
31. Wilson, N., Vickers, H., Taylor, G., and Silverman, M., Objective test for food sensitivity in asthmatic children: increased bronchial activity after cola drinks, *Br. Med. J.,* 284, 1226, 1982.
32. Munro, J. A. et al., Food allergy in migraine. Study of dietary exclusion and RAST, *Lancet,* 2, 1, 1980.
33. Egger, J., Carter, C. M., Wilson, J., Turner, M. W., and Soothill, J. F., Is migraine food allergy? A double-blind controlled trial of iligoantigenic diet treatment, *Lancet,* 2, 865, 1983.
34. Lancet (Leading article), Feingold's regimen for hyperkinesis, *Lancet,* 2, 617, 1979.
35. Feingold, B., *Why Your Child Is Hyperactive,* Random House, New York, 1975.
36. Warner, J. O. and Hathaway, M. A., The allergic basis of Meadow's syndrome, *Arch. Dis. Child.,* in press.
37. Meadow, R., Munchausen syndrome by proxy, *Arch. Dis. Child.,* 57, 92, 1982.
38. Lessof, M. H., Wraith, D. G., Merrett, T. G., Merrett, J., and Buisseret, P. D., Food allergy and intolerance in 100 patients in local and systemic effects, *Q. J. Med.,* 49, 259, 1980.
39. May, C. D., Objective clinical and laboratory studies of immediate hypersensitivity reactions to foods in asthmatic children, *J. Allergy Clin. Immunol.,* 58, 500, 1976.
40. Avery Jones, F., Commentary on alimentary symptoms (Lettsonian Lectures), *Trans. Med. Soc. London,* 81, 1964.
41. Klein, N. C., Hargrove, R. L., Sleisinger, M. D., and Jeffries, G., Eosinophilic gastroenteritis, *Medicine (Baltimore),* 49, 299, 1970.
42. Rosenkrans, P. C. M., Meijer, C. J. L. M., Van der Wal, A. M., and Lindeman, J., Allergic proctitis, a clinical and pathological entity, *Gut,* 21, 1017, 1980.
43. Sandberg, D. H., McIntosh, R. M., Bernstein, C. W., Carr, R., and Strauss, J. C., Severe steroid-responsive nephrosis associated with hypersensitivity, *Lancet,* 1, 388, 1977.
44. Whitfield, M. F. and Barr, D. G. D., Cow's milk allergy in the syndrome of thrombocytopenia with absent radius, *Arch. Dis. Child.,* 51, 337, 1976.
45. Bentley, S. J., Pearson, D. J., and Rix, K. J. B., Food hypersensitivity in irritable bowel syndrome, *Lancet,* 2, 295, 1983.
46. Jones, V. A., McLaughlan, P., Shorthouse, M., Workman, E., and Hunter, J. O., Food intolerance: a major factor in the pathogenesis of irritable bowel syndrome, *Lancet,* 2, 1115, 1982.
47. Levitt, M. D., Lasser, R. B., Schwartz, J. S., and Bond, J. H., Studies of a flatulent patient, *N. Engl. J. Med.,* 295, 260, 1976.
48. Levitt, M. D., Berggren, T., Hastings, J., and Bond, J. H., Hydrogen (H^2) catabolism in the colon of the rat, *Clin. Med.,* 84, 163, 1974.
49. Maulitz, R. M., Pratt, D. S., and Schocket, A. L., Exercise induced anaphylactic reaction to shellfish, *J. Allergy Clin. Immunol.,* 63, 633, 1979.
50. Kidd, J. M., III, Cohen, S. H., Sosman, A. J., and Fink, J. N., Food-dependent exercise-induced anaphylaxis, *J. Allergy Clin. Immunol.,* 71, 407, 1983.
51. Hanington, E., Migraine, in *Clinical Reactions to Food,* Lessof, M. H., Ed., John Wiley & Sons, Chichester, 1983, 155.
52. Blau, J. N. and Pyke, D. A., Effect of diabetes on migraine, *Lancet,* 2, 241, 1970.
53. Blau, J. N., Migraine prodromes separated from the aura: complete migraine, *Br. Med. J.,* 281, 658, 1980.
54. Faller, J. and Fox, I. H., Evidence for increased urate production by activation of adenine nucleotide turnover, *N. Engl. J. Med.,* 307, 1598, 1982.
55. MacLachlan, M. J. and Rodnan, G. P., Effects of food, fast and alcohol on serum uric acid and acute attacks of gout, *Am. J. Med.,* 42, 38, 1967.
56. Akinyanju, O. O. and Odusote, K. A., Cause of red suya syndrome in food dye orange-RN, *Lancet,* 2, 1314, 1983.
57. Ratner, D., Oren, B., and Vigder, K., Chronic dietary anticholinesterase poisoning, *Isr. J. Med. Sci.,* 19, 810, 1983.
58. Finn, R. and Cohen, H. N., 'Food allergy': fact or fiction?, *Lancet,* 1, 426, 1978.
59. Greden, J. F., Anxiety or caffeinism: a diagnostic dilemma, *Am. J. Psychiatr.,* 131, 1089, 1974.

60. Turnberg, L. A., Coffee and the gastrointestinal tract, *Gastroenterology,* 75, 529, 1978.
61. Lutz, E. G., Restless legs, anxiety and caffeinism, *Psychiatry,* 39, 693, 1978.
62. Moneret-Vautrin, D. A., False food allergies: non-specific reactions to foodstuffs, in *Clinical Reactions to Food,* Lessof, M. H., Ed., John Wiley & Sons, Chichester, 1983, 135.
63. Price, S. F., Smithson, K. W., and Castell, D. O., Food sensitivity in reflex oesophagitis, *Gastroenterology,* 75, 240, 1978.
64. Allen, D. H. and Baker, C. J., Asthma and MSG, *Med. J. Aust.,* 2, 576, 1981.
65. Bleumink, E., Allergy and nutrition, *Voeding,* 27, 593, 1966.
66. Bleumink, E., Food allergy. The chemical nature of the substances eliciting symptoms, *World Rev. Nutr. Diet.,* 12, 505, 1970.
67. Martin, C. R. A., Skin manifestations of food allergies, *Br. Food J.,* 84, 41, 1982.
68. Rice, S. L., Eitenmiller, R. R., and Koehler, P. E., Biologically active amines in food: a review, *J. Milk Food Technol.,* 39, 353, 1976.
69. Taylor, S. L., Leatherwood, M., and Lieber, E. R., A survey of histamine levels in sausages, *J. Food Prot.,* 41, 634, 1978.
70. Anon., Fish poisoning (editorial), *Br. Med. J.,* 281, 890, 1980.
71. Gilbert, R. J., Hobbs, G., Murray, C. K., Cruickshank, J. G., and Young, S. E. J., Scombrotoxic fish poisoning: features of the first 50 incidents to be reported in Britain (1976—9), *Br. Med. J.,* 281, 71, 1980.
72. Arnold, S. H. and Brown, W. D., Histamine (?) toxicity from fish products, *Adv. Food Res.,* 24, 113, 1978.
73. Garay, R. P., Daghar, G., Pernollet, M. G., Devynck, D. A., and Meyer, P., Inherited defect in a Na^+, K^+ co-transport system in erythrocytes from essential hypertensive patients, *Nature,* 284, 281, 1980.
74. Freedman, S. O., Siddiqi, A. I., Krupey, J. H., and Sehon, A. H., Identification of a simple chemical compound (chlorogenic acid) as an allergen in plant materials causing human atopic disease, *Am. J. Med. Sci.,* 244, 548, 1962.
75. Nater, J. P. and Zwartz, J. A., Atopic allergic reactions due to raw potato, *J. Allergy,* 40, 202, 1967.
76. Fries, J. H. and Glazer, I., Studies on the antigenicity of banana, raw and dehydrated, *J. Allergy,* 21, 169, 1950.
77. Perlman, F., Food allergy and vegetable proteins, *Food Technol.,* 20, 1438, 1966.
78. Coca, A. F., *Familial Non-Reaginic Food Allergy,* Charles C Thomas, Springfield, Ill., 1942.
79. Amlot, P., Personal communication, 1984.
80. Committee on Provocative Food Testing, *Ann. Allergy,* 31, 375, 1973.
81. Breneman, J. C., Hurst, A., Heiner, D., Leney, F. L., Morris, D., and Josephson, B. M., Final report of the Food Allergy Committee of the American College of Allergists on the clinical evaluation of sublingual provocative testing method for diagnosis of food allergy, *Ann. Allergy,* 33, 164, 1974.
82. Lehman, C. W., A double-blind study of sublingual provocative food testing: a study of its efficacy, *Ann. Allergy,* 45, 144, 1980.
83. Barnetson, R. St. C. and Lessof, M. H., Challenges to medical orthodoxy, in *Clinical Reactions to Food,* Lessof, M. H., Ed., John Wiley & Sons, Chichester, 1983, 15.
84. Black, A. P., A new diagnostic method in allergic disease, *Pediatrics,* 17, 716, 1956.
85. Lehman, C. W., The leukocytic food allergy test: a study of its reliability and reproducibility. Effect of diet and sublingual food drops on this test, *Ann. Allergy,* 45, 150, 1980.
86. Ferriman, A., Clinic fails its own allergy test, *Observer,* 1983.
87. Benveniste, J., The human basophil degranulation test as an *in vitro* method for the diagnosis of allergies, *Clin. Allergy,* 11, 1, 1981.

Chapter 7

INTOLERANCE TO FOOD COLORS AND OTHER ADDITIVES

Klara Miller

TABLE OF CONTENTS

I. Introduction 86

II. Tartrazine 86

III. Tartrazine and Aspirin ASA Intolerance 87

IV. Other Food Colors 88

V. Benzoates and Other Preservatives 89

VI. Food Flavors 91

VII. Frequency of Adverse Reactions 92

VIII. Basic Mechanisms 93

IX. Susceptibility 94

X. Conclusion 95

References 95

I. INTRODUCTION

The clinical symptoms of food intolerance have been described in detail in the previous chapter, and it is clear that the mechanisms involved in both allergic and nonallergic adverse responses to ingested material are complex, interdependant on other factors, and not well understood. A steadily increasing number of reports have also associated ingestion of chemicals used to color, flavor, or preserve foods, drugs, and cosmetics with the symptoms characteristic of food intolerance.

Intolerance to food additives occurs in both atopic and nonatopic subjects,[1] although as with allergic reactions to food, certain predisposing factors may be operative in atopics. For example, in a clinical study of children with allergic reactions to fish characterized by asthma and urticaria, the majority of children were found to have multiple allergies and reacted to inhaled material such as house dust, pollen, and fungi.[2] At least 10% of children under the age of 6 with asthma, rhinitis, and atopic dermatitis show clinical symptoms after challenge with food,[3] and similarly asthmatic children show an increased incidence of tartrazine sensitivity.[4] Patients with hay fever and asthma have various food hypersensitivities,[5] drawing attention to the importance of ingested agents in increasing bronchial hyperreactivity. Altered bronchial reactivity has been reported in 14 of 504 patients with asthma or rhinitis challenged with tartrazine.[6] Individuals who are intolerant to aspirin (acetylsalicylic acid [ASA]), also tend to be allergic to foods,[7] again suggesting that immune mechanisms or activation of pharmacological mediators may differ in susceptible individuals compared to those with no history of allergy. Indeed, patients with food intolerance symptoms due to nonspecific histamine response to foods eaten in relatively large amounts[8] are described as being sensitive to trace amounts of chemicals, such as insecticides, coloring dyes, and preservatives, whether they be in the food or in the environment. The susceptible individual may thus be exposed through ingestion, inhalation or external contact to a large number of chemicals which could be said to create opportunities for a wide range of adverse effects.

II. TARTRAZINE

The main chemicals associated with intolerance to additives are dyes such as tartrazine, preservatives such as benzoates or antioxidants, and flavoring agents. Tartrazine (FD & C yellow No. 5; E102) is the color most frequently implicated in food-intolerance reports, although some allowance must be made for the selective usage of the colors as well as for the frequency of testing for responses to other synthetic colors in clinical trials.

Tartrazine is an azo-based dye, yellow in color, and present in a great variety of foods, soft drinks, and medicines where it may be present in coatings, shells, or excipient material. Tartrazine and most compounds used in the formulation of drugs have been selected because of their toxicoligical clearance for "safety in use" as food additives. While tartrazine and other synthetic colors have been extensively tested, specific regulations on food colors vary considerably between countries, so that some colors can be considered safe and acceptable in one country but prohibited in another.[9]

The majority of reports on tartrazine intolerance involve pharmaceutical preparations containing the dye. The first report of intolerance to tartrazine was of three patients, each of whom reacted to a corticosteroid preparation containing the coloring.[10] One of the patients was being treated for severe bronchial asthma, one was suffering from collagen disease and had a history of intolerance to ASA, and the third was known to react violently to drugs of mercurial or coal tar origin. It is evident in this first report that the patients suffered from preexisting disorders and were also intolerant to drugs and chemicals other than tartrazine, suggesting multiple susceptibilities to chemicals. This relationship between ASA intolerance and intolerance to tartrazine as well as other substances will be discussed later in the chapter.

During the 1960s and 1970s, reports of about 25 patients reacting to the tartrazine content of drug products were published. For example, Chafee and Settipane[11] clearly incriminated tartrazine as a cause of asthmatic attacks in a woman on drug therapy. Withdrawal of the drug brought relief, but coughing and wheezing were noted after challenge tests with tartrazine-colored vitamin tablets. The report by Feingold[12] that imbibed soft drinks containing tartrazine caused allergic symptoms in children focused attention on the use of azo dyes in food as well as drug products.

Dr. Feingold further claimed that behavior disorders in children were due to an inborn chemical reaction affecting the nervous system of certain genetically predisposed individuals and that synthetic food colors and flavors as well as salicylates were the causative agents. Recent data evaluating the relationship between hyperactivity, salicylates, artificial food colors, and flavors indicate that the symptoms of the vast majority of hyperactive children are not related to additives in their diet.[13,14] On present evidence it seems that hyperkinesis, or hyperactivity, cannot be considered a disease or a syndrome, but is in fact a symptom with a variety of causes which need to be treated by a multidisciplinary cooperative effort involving the home, school, and family doctor.[15]

The controversy over the use of elimination diets designed to be low in salicylates and free of food additives[16] has focused attention on the amount of tartrazine that is ingested in food such as cheese, juice, pickles, sweets, and cake mixes. At present, however, the ingestion of tartrazine and the clinical manifestations of urticaria and asthma appear only to have been clearly demonstrated in highly selected groups of patients, and there is little evidence to substantiate the claim that tartrazine is capable of inducing intolerance in a healthy subject.

III. TARTRAZINE AND ASPIRIN ASA INTOLERANCE

Adverse reactions to tartrazine occur most commonly in subjects who are sensitive to ASA. Between 10 and 40% of ASA-sensitive patients, depending on the test protocol followed, respond to tartrazine with reactions ranging from severe asthma to urticaria and mild rhinitis.[1,17,18] Before discussing this population, it might be appropriate to consider more generally the effect of ASA ingestion.

It is now well establihsed that ASA and other nonsteroidal analgesics inhibit the prostaglandin synthesis system via the cyclooxygenase pathway.[19,20] The inhibition of prostaglandins is associated with the release of histamine and other vasoactive mediators from mast cells. An increase in plasma histamine levels has been demonstrated during adverse responses to ASA induced in vivo during clinical studies.[21] In addition, other studies where plasma concentrations of prostaglandin have been measured during the onset of clinical reactions to ASA have shown significantly reduced concentrations of PGF_2 though not of PGE_2,[22] suggesting an ASA-induced alteration in the balance between the various prostanoid metabolites rather than a total inhibition of cyclooxygenase pathways. Indeed, the recent finding that blood prostaglandin levels may be abnormal in ASA-intolerant individuals[23] implies an inherent defect of prostaglandin metabolism which could be triggered by both pharmacological or allergic reactions.

However, while enhanced histamine release in vitro has been reported with lipoxygenase metabolites[24] as well as with inhibitors of the cyclooxygenase pathway,[25] leukocytes from ASA-intolerant donors when stimulated with A23187 and/or ASA do not release in vitro more histamine than leukocytes from normal controls.[26] Thus there is little evidence at present of a link between the onset of symptoms of ASA intolerance, arachidonic acid metabolites, and histamine release.

ASA has also been shown to inhibit prostaglandin synthesis in the gastric mucosa,[27] increasing the permeability of the gastroepithelial membrane and permitting the absorption of molecules too large to cross the mucosal barrier under normal conditions.[28] This effect is thought to lead to the amplification of immediate hypersensitivity reactions to food components in animals such as the guinea pig.[29] A similar effect has been observed in a boy with local symptoms of hypersensitivity to peanuts who developed a life-threatening asthma attack after concomitant ingestion of peanuts and ASA.[30] The sequence of events was identical to those demonstrated in animal experiments and suggests that ASA, though causing increased absorption of macromolecules, may potentiate the effect of food allergens in asthmatics.

On the other hand ASA may cause an improvement in asthma,[31] and this again supports the hypothesis that the balance between different arachidonic acid metabolites may differ in normal, ASA-tolerant and ASA-intolerant asthmatic individuals. The familial nature of some cases of both ASA and tartrazine intolerance[32-34] underlies the need for future research into possible inborn or acquired errors of metabolism which might be involved in adverse reactions to some chemicals.

It must be emphasized that no effects of tartrazine on the prostaglandin pathways have been observed.[35,36] This is not an unexpected finding, as was tartrazine to inhibit cyclooxygenase pathways; the cross-reactivity between tartrazine and ASA ought to have occurred much more commonly. Nevertheless, while susceptibility to tartrazine may occur in the absence of ASA intolerance, the great majority of reported cases are ASA-sensitive individuals. Whether ASA and/or tartrazine may exacerbate a preexisting intolerance caused by natural salicylates in the diet is not known. Salicylates are present in a number of vegetables and fruits, notably peas, rhubarb, bananas, and grapes. Many of the natural salicylates are stable and appear unchanged in food products such as preserves and wine.[37] A range of synthetic salicylates are also used to flavor sweets, ice cream, soft drinks, and cake mixes. The chemical similarity of these materials with ASA as well as other chemicals poses a possible explanation for the multiple susceptibility to other substances seen in ASA-sensitive patients.

There is an obvious need for studies on the influence of ASA and tartrazine on pharmacological mediator release or formation in normal and intolerant individuals. A possible relationship between prostaglandin and a slow-reacting substance of anaphylaxis (SRS-A) has been suggested,[38] indicating that alterations in arachidonic acid metabolic pathways may be important. The potential role of SRS-A as a mediator of intolerant reactions has not yet been investigated. All that can be said at present is that a substantial proportion of ASA-sensitive individuals do react to tartrazine and that intolerance to tartrazine does not appear to be mediated by inhibition of prostaglandin synthesis or IgE production.

IV. OTHER FOOD COLORS

Tartrazine differs from other azo dyes in that it is not metabolized by specific azoreductase enzymes in the liver, and this has led to the suggestion that it may not possess a true azo link[39] but exists rather as a keto-hydrazine tautomer (Figure 1). Whatever the case, there are close similarities between the pyrazol and sulfophenyl portions characteristic of the tartrazine molecule and the molecular structure of the other synthetic food colors (Figure 2). It is not surprising therefore that several clinical studies have demonstrated cross-reactivity or multiple reactivity to a wide range of food colors. In one study, subjects were tested with amaranth, sunset yellow FCF, and ponceau 4R, and while no definite patterns for the reaction to the different azo colors were seen, 27

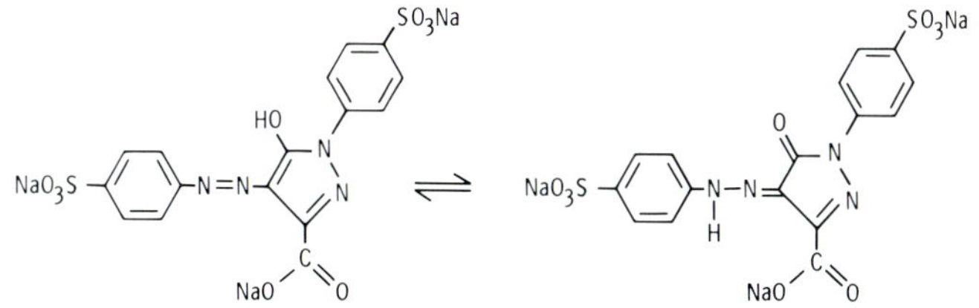

FIGURE 1. General structure of tartrazine.

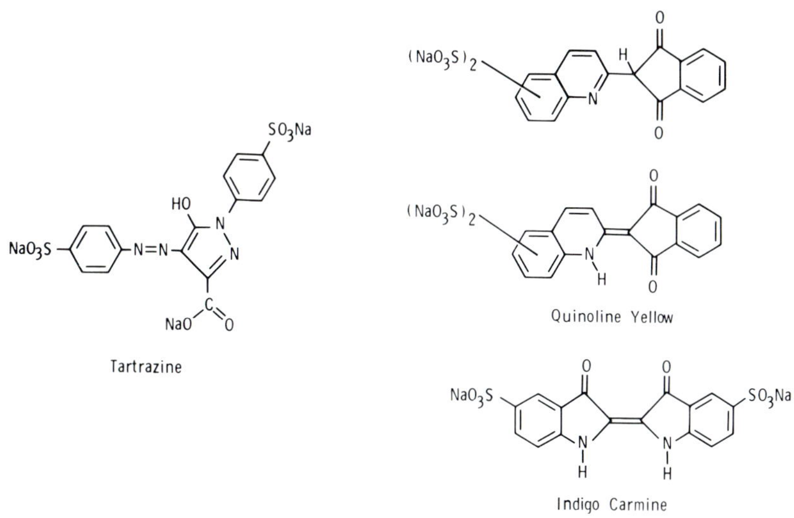

FIGURE 2. Structural comparison of tartrazine and nonazo dyes.

patients reacted to some azo dyes at dosages similar to those applied for tartrazine.[40] Patients with chronic urticaria who have been tested for their responses to a wide range of food colors also showed positive reactions to erythrosine (a nonazo dye), and as many as 26% reacted to the natural food color annatto.[41] In view of the known ability of naturally occurring pigments to combine with proteins, this latter observation is of considerable interest.

Various carotenoid extracts have been used as food colors for centruies.[42] Examples include the yellow color of saffron, the orange-red of paprika, and the pinkish yellow of annatto. Commercially, annatto is extracted from the seed of a small tree, *Bixa orellana L,* and the extract is used either as an oil-soluble (bixin) or a water-soluble (norbixin) pigment depending on its application (Figure 3). Usuage is mainly in dairy and fat-based products, smoked fish, cereals, and ice creams; in each case the pigment is absorbed onto the protein and carbohydrate components of the foodstuff and is not leached out by water. In view of the widespread presence of carotenoids in fruits and vegetables and the complexity of the Western diet, it would be impossible to identify whether a naturally occurring or an added component was the original offending substance.

Reactions with other dietary components must also be considered in the case of food-intolerant individuals. Such components include preservatives such as benzoic acid and antioxidants as well as synthetic food flavorings.

V. BENZOATES AND OTHER PRESERVATIVES

Patients with respiratory disorders and ASA sensitivity may also be intolerant to

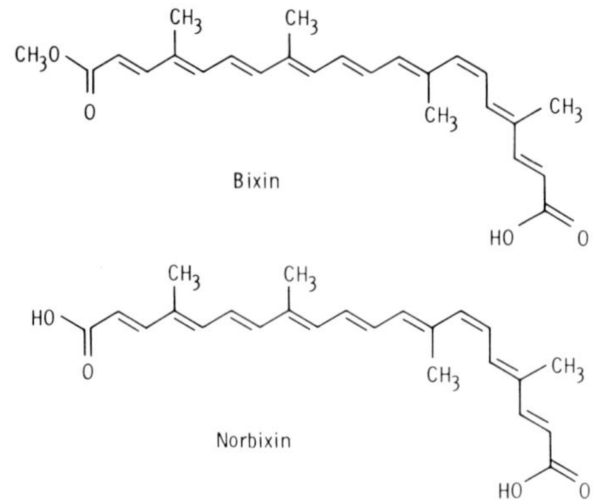

FIGURE 3. General structure of annatto.

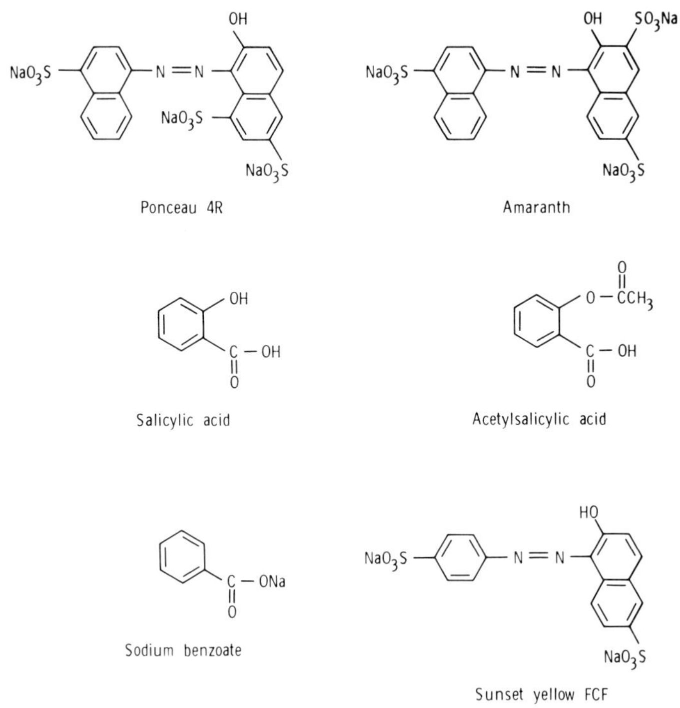

FIGURE 4. Structural comparison of cross-reactive compounds.

preservatives such as sodium benzoate and benzoate esters, widely used in different foods and beverages, and there is a close relation between intolerance to ASA and intolerance to food colors and benzoate preservatives. This multiple reactivity appears to be due to similar chemical structures shared by ASA, the benzoate molecule, and azo dyes (Figure 4). Whatever immunological or pharmacological mediator mechanisms may be involved, the similarity between chemical ''epitopes'' would explain why patients suffering from chronic urticaria and ASA-associated asthma often improve when put on diets free from azo colors and preservatives.[43,44]

As with salicylates, benzoates occur naturally in some foods, and in berries such as cranberries and blueberries, levels can reach a concentration of 100-mg benzoic acid per 100 g.[37] It is interesting that cross-reactivity with benzoates has been reported most often in studies carried out in Scandinavia, where eating of such berries may be more common than in other parts of the world. The possibility that susceptible individuals could develop benzoate intolerance through ingestion of foods with high natural amounts of the compound cannot be excluded. Benzoates also occur naturally in many other foods such as coffee beans, teas, and red wine, although at about one tenth of the levels found in blueberries.

Sulfiting agents have also been implicated in acute adverse reactions. Many foods and beverages contain sulfur dioxide, which is used as a preservative and antioxidant, and sulfur dioxide plays an essential role in the manufacture of beer and wine. It has been shown to induce acute exacerbation of symptoms in sensitive asthmatics.[45]

In one study, 14 asthmatic patients known to be sensitive to orange soft drink were given an aqueous solution of SO_2 in a concentration comparable to that permitted in orange drinks.[46] A rapid onset of bronchospasm was observed in eight patients. The mechanism in unknown, but it appears that dose level may be important. Sulfur dioxide and sulfiting agents may be used in situations where ordinary food labeling requirements for additives would not apply — e.g., in wine or on prepared, raw potatoes or grapes — so that sulfite might not readily be implicated in any adverse reaction.

The use of *n*-octyl gallate as an antioxidant in beer also caused concern after it was demonstrated to be a contact sensitizer. A positive reaction to a 0.1% *n*-octyl gallate solution was demonstrated in 13 out of 445 volunteers after repeated cutaneous applications.[47] Oral mucosa tests conducted using beer containing 20 ppm *n*-octyl gallate produced strong positive reactions in individuals previously sensitized by the cutaneous application of this agent, whereas nonsensitized individuals did not react. Nevertheless, it is important to point out that strong reactions were seen to occur only in "contact-sensitized" individuals, either working with or repeatedly challenged with these agents. It is also important that in experimental animal studies the repeated ingestion of even potent contact-sensitizing agents has been shown to lead to a state of immunological tolerance[48] and that the animal is effectively protected from initiating an adverse reaction.[49] Kahn and co-workers[50] provided evidence to suggest that this could also occur with gallate esters. The experiments demonstrated that guinea pigs previously exposed by the oral route failed to react when the same material was subsequently administered by injection. These observations taken together with the results from other experimental animal studies explain the lack of recorded illness in the majority of the population but offer no explanation for the occasional reports of intolerant individuals.

Butylated hydroxytoluene (BHT) and butylated hydroxyanisole (BHA) are also widely used antioxidants and have been reported to cause urticaria and asthma in a few individuals. Interest in these agents stems from Jublin's observation that 14 to 15% of patients suffering from chronic urticaria also reacted against these additives,[41] again suggesting that indivuduals sensitive to one substance also tend to react to a variety of other substances.

VI. FOOD FLAVORS

Reactivity to food flavors is recognized in food additive-intolerant patients.[52] Peru balsam and its products have been suspect flavoring agents for many years. Peru balsam is an oleoresin obtained from *Myroxylon pereirae,* a tree which grows mainly in Central America. Crude resin extracts contain 50 to 60% cinnamein, an ester of cinnamic and benzoic acid, and approximately 28% resin, styracine, and vanillin. The balsam has had considerable use in perfumes, flavors, toilet waters, etc. Peru balsam oil is the refined form of the resin obtained after solvent extraction or distillation. The oil contains large amounts of benzyl benzoate and benzyl cinnamate. Previous sensitization with vanillin or cinnamate could explain some of the positive patch test reactions to Peru balsam seen in individuals apparently not previously exposed to this substance.[53]

Finally, it has been observed that individuals whose clinical symptoms of food intolerance are precipitated by large amounts of food are frequently sensitive to trace amounts of chemicals such as insecticides, azo dyes, and other chemicals whether they be in the food or in the environment.[54]

VII. FREQUENCY OF ADVERSE REACTIONS

The precise assessment of the frequency of food allergy, or intolerance is difficult, since diagnosis has depended largely on subjective methods associated with clinical screening tests and the interpretation of a patient's previous history (see Chapter 6). Thus widely varying estimates of prevalence may be found in the literature. It has been suggested, for example, that between 0.3 and 20% of children suffer from or have suffered from some form of dietary-intolerance disorder.[55] The wide range of incidence reflects the effects of selective bias and different diagnostic criteria employed in various studies and emphasizes the difficulty in establishing a useful estimate of prevalence.

In studies on food allergies it is possible to work with a defined population, reasonably precise clinical histories, and, in the case of milk intolerance, a defined material. When it comes to assessing the frequency of allergy or intolerance to food additives, the problem is considerably more difficult. This is because a number of colors and additives are often used in conjunction and appear in a wide variety of foodstuffs. As reactivity between structurally related colors and additives also occurs, a given individual may not know what particular a food or food component triggers the adverse reaction. Studies concerning reactivity to food additives have generally been restricted to selected populations and mainly to patients receiving services at the hospital for the treatment of "allergy-like" diseases. These studies cannot provide true estimates of prevalence, since extrapolation from responses obtained in a given selected group to prediction of responses in the general population makes the assumption that there is no difference in susceptibility associated with the underlying disorder and that any "allergic" condition is as capable as another of reflecting the likely occurrence of adverse reactions in the general population. Furthermore, such extrapolation cannot take into account the influence upon the number of positive results obtained of the phase of the underlying disease at the time of testing and the testing procedures used. It is reasonable to assume that the susceptibility of the general population is likely to be considerably less than that of the special groups studied.

Studies on selected populations, albeit under variable conditions of testing, have, however, highlighted food additives which may be responsible for syndromes of intolerance. To obtain an approximate figure for the prevalence of additives associated with exacerbation of chronic urticaria, Juhlin[41] reviewed the literature for relevant information and in conjunction with his own data reached the following conclusions. In patients with chronic urticaria 33 to 50% of individuals tested reacted to one or more food additives. Of the additives employed in the provocation tests, tartrazine produced a reaction in 5 to 46% of those tested; other azo dyes gave from 5 to 20% positives. Among the preservatives considered, benzoate derivatives produced reactions in between 3 and 44%, and the antioxidants BHT and BHA yielded an incidence of 14 to 15%. Thus even in sensitive individuals, there was a wide range of reactivity. In another study,[56] reactions to individual food colors yielded the following percentages: among 61 patients suffering from chronic urticaria and/or angioneurotic edema 11% reacted to tartrazine, 17% to sunset yellow FCF, 16% to food red 17, 9% to amaranth, 15% to ponceau 4R, 12% to erythrosine, and 14% to brilliant blue FCF. In the same study, the natural color annatto, a commonly used color in butter and edible fat products, was also studied. Challenge was performed with a dose equivalent to the amount present in 25 g of butter. In the group 26 patients reacted within about 4 hr of ingestion, indicating that natural food colors may also induce intolerance reactions at least as frequently as synthetic dyes. There was, however, no pattern of cross-reactivity between the azo dyes and the natural annatto extract. In the same study, 30% of patients reacted to ASA and 15% to sodium benzoate.

One investigation on asthmatic children reported that of 32 children studied, 1 in 3 reacted to ASA and 1 in 5 reacted to tartrazine and/or benzoates.[57] Bronchial sensitivity to histamine increased in 4 out of 10 patients with childhood asthma 30 min after tartrazine ingestion but not after a placebo.[58] Weber and colleagues[59] investigated 45 asthmatic patients and found only 3 who reacted to commonly employed color agents.[59] Although this is equivalent to an incidence of 5 to 6%, it must be emphasized that the subjects were selected to include individuals with a suggestive history of food sensitivity. A more systematic approach has been employed in a recent study undertaken in Denmark.[37] The frequency of asthma, chronic rhinitis, and chronic urticaria was assessed in the general population over 16 years of age and determined to be in the order of 3.8, 1.9, and 0.5%, respectively.[60-62] The frequency of adverse reactions to food additives within each group was then determined by reference to previous case histories and previous provocation tests. It was concluded that 0.01 to 0.1% of the general population were sensitive to both tartrazine and benzoates. These figures are in the same order as those suggested by Juhlin,[41] who estimated that in every 10 million people about 40,000 will show intolerance to ASA (0.4%), 6000 to tartrazine (0.06%), and 5000 to benzoates (0.05%). In France, sensitivity to tartrazine was estimated to be between 0.03[63] and 0.15%.[64] The range is obviously very wide, is based on the incidence in only one group (asthmatics), and ignores the possible international differences in the incidence of asthma and its causes. Nevertheless, these figures suggest that tartrazine-intolerant individuals may be numbered at least as 1 in 10,000.[65]

VIII. BASIC MECHANISMS

There is no evidence at present that adverse reactions to tartrazine or other additives are mediated through specific immunoglobulin E (IgE) antibodies normally implicated in type I allergic reactions.

The majority of chemicals used as food dyes are of low molecular weight and would therefore be expected to act as haptens, inducing an immune response only after binding to a serum or tissue protein. A number of animal studies have shown that tartrazine, the major dye to be investigated, exhibits relatively little protein-binding capacity in comparison with other nonazo dyes.[66] Ingestion of tartrazine, however, results in the appearance of metabolic products in the urine and feces.[67] Tartrazine is now known to be metabolized by cecal bacteria to yield a variety of reaction products, some of which are thought to be capable of interacting with proteins to form associated conjugates.[68]

Conjugated tartrazine preparations can induce specific IgG antibodies after parenteral administration to rabbits.[69] These antibodies were shown to cross-react extensively with *p*-azobenzenesulfonate.[70] Further studies into the ability of various food dyes to inhibit the interaction between the tartrazine-specific antibody and the sulfonate demonstrated that tartrazine, sunset yellow, and amaranth all inhibited this reaction, whereas brilliant blue, sulfanilate, and ASA had no effect. Such studies emphasize that the chemical structure of the tartrazine molecule has features similar to those of benzoates and other azo compounds and, by inference, imply that some degree of cross-reactivity is likely to occur between all azo dyes. The demonstration that a tartrazine conjugate is immunogenic when injected and gives rise to a normal humoral response in an animal model does not imply that it can provoke an allergic response in man.

A recent study, however, has demonstrated the production of a tartrazine specific reaginic antibody in a rat model.[71] In this study the parenterally administered tartrazine, covalently coupled to ovalbumin, was presented in association with carrageenan. The induction of reaginic antibody to tartrazine was dependent on the particular adjuvant properties of carrageenan. The response could be enhanced by a secondary challenge but declined rapidly and thereafter could not be reelicited. Suppressor T (T_s) lymphocytes are thought to control the experimental induction of reaginic antibody,[72] and animal models such as the one described above might provide some insight as to whether tartrazine under certain conditions could bypass the normal regulatory mechanisms. While there have been reports of low levels of T_s cells in atopic disease states,[73] there is nothing, however, to suggest that protein-tartrazine conjugates would give rise to IgE production in these individuals. Furthermore, the covalently bound material is not representative of human exposure, as spontaneous covalent binding between tartrazine and albumin appears to be weak.[74]

An association between clinically identified intolerance to tartrazine and an antigen-specific IgD antibody has been reported.[75] Little is known of the functional properties of circulting IgD, although elevated IgD antibodies have been reported in certain allergic states.[76,77] The specificity of the IgD antitartrazine antibodies found in the above-mentioned study was to the sulfophenyl portion of the tartrazine molecule, and the azo and pyrazol portions of the molecule were found not to participate as antigenic determinants. The majority of the tartrazine-sensitive patients also had high total-serum IgE levels, indicative of allergies to a variety of substances. Whether humoral immunological mechanisms other than those commonly involved in drug and food allergy play a role in adverse reactions to food additives, particularly in hypersensitive individuals, can only be clarified by further investigations.

Tartrazine is apparently able to induce delayed type hypersensitivity reactions in the guinea pig,[78] suggesting that tartrazine contains hapten determinants eliciting lymphocyte-mediated reactivity. While there is no evidence that this finding is related to the clinical signs of tartrazine-induced intolerance, it is nevertheless of interest. It is known, for example, that benzoates added to many foodstuffs as preservatives may give rise to exacerbations of eczema in individuals who have a delayed type hypersensitivity reaction to compounds of comparable chemical structure present in cosmetics, pharmaceuticals, and topically applied medicaments.[79] In addition, food components such as nickel, chromates, and some aromatic compounds used as fragrances or flavors may act as contact sensitizers and then cause contact dermatitis after oral ingestion.[37] It is estimated that 8000 women per million of the Danish population have recurrence of attacks of hand eczema from nickel compounds present in the food.[80] While nickel allergy may be a very specific problem, it demonstrates that various mechanisms and pathways may be involved in inducing intolerance to a low-molecular weight compound.

IX. SUSCEPTIBILITY

It would appear that genetic factors may predispose individuals to a number of diseases, and this may also hold true for certain food-intolerance syndromes. There are, for example, suggestive links between the HLA haplotype A1/B8 and atopic eczema[81] and between HLA B8/DW3 and gluten sensitivity.[82] A recent study of ASA-sensitive asthmatics, however, has failed to show any statistically significant increase in any known DR antigen or any correlation with A or B locus typing.[83] Most studies of genetic factors relating to host susceptibility have not yet demonstrated convincing associations with increased frequency of specific HLA antigens. This failure may perhaps be due to the paucity of evidence so far accumulated.[84] However, even in ankylosing spondylitis (where the association between HLA and disease is convincing), 10% of Caucasian patients presenting the disease lack the diagnostic B27 antigen. Indeed, recent experimental evidence suggests that there may well exist a whole class of non-HLA-linked genes that also control immune responses to foreign substances.[85] Until these areas have been explored, genetic testing for susceptibility to ingested materials remains of only restricted value.

Genetic factors can only come into play following the appropriate exposure to the environmental stimulus. Developmental and/or environmental pressures must be superimposed upon a genetic predisposition before a state of intolerance can appear. A predisposition to dietary intolerance is obviously a real phenomenon, but at this point we remain unclear as to how this operates.

X. CONCLUSION

There is little doubt that intolerance to food additives occurs in a minority of the population. These individuals generally appear to belong to a select group that exhibit multiple reactivity to a variety of ingested and inhaled material. Whether food colors or other food additives are able to initiate a state of intolerance in susceptible individuals or whether they act only on previously affected individuals can only be resolved by further research into the epidemiological and scientific aspects of food intolerance.

It must be emphasized that there is at present no suitable experimental model available to assess the possible allergic potential of new food additives. Furthermore, the mechanisms for production of adverse reactions to food additives have not been demonstrated to have those immunological components usually associated with hypersensitivity reactions, thus stressing the need to explore other possible mechanisms for modulating the immune response as well as investigating the role of pharmacological mediators. At present, for those individuals who do react adversely to food additives there is a need for better access to information on what ingredients of both natural and synthetic origin are present in their food products and medications.

REFERENCES

1. **Stenuis, B. S. M. and Lemola, M.**, Hypersensitivity to acetylsalicylic acid (ASA) and tartrazine in patients with asthma, *Clin. Allergy*, 6, 119, 1976.
2. **Aas, K.**, Studies of hypersensitivity to fish — a clinical study, *Int. Arch. Allergy*, 29, 346, 1966.
3. **Gonzalez de la Reguera, I., Inigo, J. F., and Gehling, A.**, The importance of food sensitization in atropic dermatities, *Dermatologica*, 143, 288, 1971.
4. **Hariparsad, D., Wilson, N., Dixon, C., and Scherman, M.**, Oral tartrazine challenge in childhood asthma: effect on bronchial reactivity, *Clin. Allergy*, 14, 81, 1984.
5. **Erickson, N. E.**, Food sensitivity reported by patients with asthma and hay fever, *Allergy*, 33, 189, 1978.
6. **Rosenhall, L.**, Evaluation of intolerance to analgesics, preservatives and food colorants with challenge tests, *Eur. J. Respir. Dis.*, 63, 410, 1982.
7. **Speer, F.**, Aspirin allergy: a clinical study, *South. Med. J.*, 68, 314, 1975.
8. **Moneret-Vautrin, D. A.**, in *The Mast Cell — Its Role in Health and Disease*, Pepys, J. and Edwards, A. M., Eds., Pitman Medical, Tunbridge Wells, U. K., 1979, 431.
9. **Parker, L. E.**, Regulatory approaches to food coloration, in *Developments in Food Colours*, Vol. 2, Walford, J., Ed., Elsevier Applied Science, London, 1983, chap. 1.
10. **Lockey, S. D.**, Allergic reactions due to FD & C yellow no. 5 tartrazine, an aniline dye used as a coloring and identifying agent in various steroids, *Ann. Allergy*, 17, 719, 1959.

11. Chafee, F. H. and Settipane, G. A., Asthma caused by FD and C approved dyes, *J. Allergy,* 40, 65, 1967.
12. Feingold, B. F., Food additives and child development, *Hosp. Pract.,* 8, 11, 1973.
13. Stare, F. J., Whelan, E. M., and Sheridan, M., Diet and hyperactivity: is there a relationship?, *Pediatrics,* 66, 521, 1980.
14. Mattes, J. A. and Gittelman, R., Effects of artificial food colorings in children with hyperactive symptoms. A critical review and results of a controlled study, *Arch. Gen. Psychiatr.,* 38, 714, 1981.
15. American Academy of Allergy and Immunology and National Institute of Allergy and Infectious Diseases Report. Adverse Reactions to Foods, Natl. Inst. Health Publ. 84-2442, 1984.
16. Conners, C. K., Goyette, C. H., and Southwick, D. A., Food additives and hyperkinesis: a preliminary report of a double-blind crossover experiment, *Psychopharmacol. Bull.,* 12, 10, 1976.
17. Settipane, G. A., Chafee, F. H., Postman, I. M., Levine, M. I., Saken, J. H., Barrick, R. M., Nicholas, S. S., Schwartz, H. J., Honsiger, R. W., and Klein, D. E., Significance of tartrazine sensitivity in chronic urticaria of unknown aetiology, *J. Allergy Clin. Immunol.,* 57, 541, 1976.
18. Vedanthan, P. K., Menon, M. M., Ball, T. D., and Bergini, D., Aspirin and tartrazine oral challenge: incidence of adverse reponse in chronic childhood asthma, *J. Allergy Clin. Immunol.,* 60, 8, 1977.
19. Vane, J. R., Inhibition of prostaglandin synthesis as a mechanism of action for aspirin like drugs, *Nature (London) New Biol.,* 231, 232, 1971.
20. Szczeklik, A., Gryglewski, R. J., and Czerniawska-Mysik, G., Relationship of inhibition of prostaglandin biosynthesis by analgesics to asthma attacks in aspirin-sensitive patients, *Br. Med. J.,* i, 67, 1975.
21. Stevenson, D. D., Arroyare, C. M., Ohat, K. N., and Tan, E. M., Oral aspirin challenge in asthmatic patients: a study of plasma histamine, *Clin. Allergy,* 6, 493, 1973.
22. Assad, S. I., Youlten, L. J. F., and Lessof, M. H., Specific desensitizaiton in "aspirin-sensitive" urticaria; plasma prostaglandin levels and clinical manifestations, *Clin. Allergy,* 13, 459, 1983.
23. Assad, S. I., Kemeny, D. M., Youlten, L. J. F., Frankland, A. W., and Lessof, M. H., Effect of aspirin in "aspirin sensitive" patients, *Br. Med. J.,* 288, 745, 1984.
24. Peters, S. P., Kagey-Sobotka, A., MacGlashan, D., Jr., Siegel, M. C., and Lichenstein, L. H., The modulation of human basophil histamine release by products of the 5-lipoxygenase pathway, *J. Immunol.,* 129, 796, 1982.
25. Wojanr, R. J., Hearn, T., and Starkweather, S., Augmentation of allergic histamine release from human leukocytes by nonsteroidal anti-inflammatory analgesic agents, *J. Allergy Clin. Immunol.,* 66, 37, 1980.
26. Bochner, B. S., Thomas, L. L., Godnik, L., and Samter, M., Effect of the calcium inophore A23187 and aspirin on histamine release in vitro from leukocytes of aspirin-intolerant donors, *Int. Arch. Allergy Appl. Immunol.,* 74, 104, 1984.
27. Whittle, B. J. R., Higgs, G. A., Eakins, K. E., Moncada, S., and Vane, J. R., Selective inhibition of prostaglandin production in inflammatory exudates and gastric mucosa, *Nature,* 284, 271, 1980.
28. Wood, J. G. and Davenport, H. W., Measurement of canine gastric permeability to plasma proteins in normal and protein losing states, *Gastroenterology,* 82, 725, 1982.
29. Flemström, G., Marsden, N. V. B., and Richter, W., Passive cutaneous anaphylaxis in guinea pigs elicited by gastric absorption of dextran induced by acetylsalicylic acid, *Int. Arch. Allergy Appl. Immunol.,* 51, 627, 1976.
30. Cant, A. J., Gibson, P., and Dancy, M., Food hypersensitivity made life threatening by ingestion of aspirin, *Br. Med. J.,* 288, 755, 1984.
31. Szceklik, A. and Nizankowska, E., Asthma improved by aspirin-like drugs, *Br. J. Dis. Chest,* 77, 153, 1983.
32. Lockey, R. F., Rucknagel, D. L., and Vanselow, N. A., Familial occurrence of asthma, nasal polyps and aspirin intolerance, *Ann. Intern. Med.,* 78, 57, 1973.
33. Thurton, C. W. G., Morris, L., Buckingham, J. A., Lawler, S. D., and Turner-Warwick, M., Histocompatibility antigens in asthma: population and family studies, *Thorax,* 34, 670, 1979.
34. Settipane, G. A. and Pudupakkam, R. K., Aspirin intolerance. III. Subtypes, familial occurrence and cross-reactivity with tartrazine, *J. Allergy Clin. Immun.,* 56, 215, 1975.
35. Gerber, J. G., Payne, N. A., Oelz, O., Nies, A. S., and Oates, J. A., Tartrazine and the prostaglandin system, *J. Allergy Clin. Immunol.,* 63, 289, 1979.
36. Vargraftig, B. B., Bessot, J. C., and Pauli, G., Is tartrazine-induced asthma related to inhibition of prostaglandin biosynthesis?, *Respiration,* 39, 276, 1980.
37. Poulsen, E., Danish report on allergy and intolerance to food ingredients and food additives, Toxicology Forum, Aspen, Colorado, 1980.
38. Mathe, A. A., Strandberg, K., and Yen, S.-S., Prostaglandin release by slow-reacting substance from guinea pig and human lung tissue, *Prostaglandins,* 14, 1105, 1977.
39. Wright, S. E., Food additives research project report, *Aust. Food Manuf.,* 32, 32, 1963.

40. Michaelsson, G. and Juhlin, L., Urticaria induced by preservatives and dye additives in food and drugs, *Br. J. Dermatol.*, 88, 525, 1973.
41. Juhlin, L., Recurrent urticaria: clinical investigation of 330 patients, *Br. J. Dermatol.*, 104, 369, 1981.
42. Counsell, J. N., Some synthetic carotenoids as food colours, in *Developments in Food Colours*, Vol. 1, Walford, J., Ed., Elsevier Applied Science, London, 1980, chap. 6.
43. Ros, A., Juhlin, L., and Michaelsson, G., A follow-up study of patients with recurrent urticaria and hypersensitivity to aspirin, benzoates and dyes, *Br. J. Dermatol.*, 95, 19, 1976.
44. Douglas, H. M. G., Dietary treatment of patients with chronic urticaria and intolerance to aspirin and food additives, *Br. J. Dermatol.*, 93, 135, 1975.
45. Freedman, B. J., Sulphur dioxide in foods and beverages — its use as a preservative and its effect on asthma, *Br. J. Dis. Chest*, 128, 1980.
46. Freedman, B. J., Asthma induced by sulphur dioxide benzoate and tartrazine contained in orange drinks, *Clin. Allergy*, 407, 1977.
47. Report IBT F9655, IBT P8473 and IBT No. 8473, Industrial Biotest Laboratories, Illinois, 1971.
48. Chase, M. W., Inhibition of experimental drug allergy by prior feeding of the sensitising agent, *Proc. Soc. Exp. Biol. Med.*, 61, 257, 1946.
49. Challacombe, S. J. and Tomasi, T. I., Systemic tolerance and secretory immunity after oral immunisation, *J. Exp. Med.*, 152, 1459, 1980.
50. Kahn, G., Pharnuphak, P., and Claman, H. N., Propyl gallate-contact sensitization and orally-induced tolerance, *Arch. Dermatol.*, 109, 506, 1974.
51. Fisherman, E. W. and Cohen, G. N., Aspirin and other cross-reacting small chemicals in known aspirin intolerant patients, *Ann. Allergy*, 31, 476, 1973.
52. August, P. J., Urticaria. Diagnostic methods and criteria, in *Proc. 1st Food Allergy Workshop*, Medical Education Services, Oxford, 1980, 76.
53. Rothenborg, H. W., Occupational dermatitis in beekeeper exposed to poplar resins in beeswax, *Arch. Dermatol.*, 95, 381, 1967.
54. Gerrard, J. W., The diagnosis of the food-allergic patient, in *The Mast Cell — Its Role in Health and Disease*, Pepys, J. and Edwards, A. M., Eds., Pitman Medical, Tunbridge Wells, U.K., 1979, 418.
55. Ogle, K. A. and Bullock, J. D., Children with allergic rhinitis and/or bronchial asthma treated with elimination diet, *Ann. Allergy*, 39, 8, 1977.
56. Mikkelsen, H., Larsen, J. C., and Tarding, F., Hypersensitivity reactions to food colours with special reference to the natural colour annatto extract (butter colour), *Arch. Toxicol.*, Suppl. 1, 141, 1978.
57. Syvanen, P. and Beckman, A., Abstract, *Nordic Congress of Allergology*, Munksgaard, Copenhagen, 1978, 58.
58. Hariparsad, D., Wilson, N., Dixon, C., and Silverman, M., Oral tartrazine challenge in childhood asthma: effect on bronchial reactivity, *Clin. Allergy*, 14, 81, 1984.
59. Weber, R. W., Hoffman, M., Raine, D. A., and Nelson, H. S., Incidence of bronchoconstruction due to aspirin, azo dyes, non azo dyes and preservatives in a population of perennial asthmatics, *J. Allergy Clin. Immunol.*, 64, 32, 1979.
60. Weeke, E. R., Kamper-Jorgensen, F., and Pedersen, P. A., Forkomst af overfolsomhedseksem i den voksne danske befolkning, *Ugeskr. Laeg.*, 142, 3340, 1980.
61. Weeke, E. R., Kamser-Jorgensen, F., and Pedersen, P. A., Forekomst af naeldefeber i den voksne danske befolkning, *Ugeskr. Laeg.*, 142, 3269, 1980.
62. Weeke, E. R., Kamper-Jorgensen, F., and Pedersen, P. A., Forekomst af asthma bronchiale i den voksne danske befolkning, *Ugeskr. Laeg.*, 142, 3272, 1980.
63. Moneret-Vantrin, D. A., Gulliat, J. P., and Demange, G., Allergy and intolerance to tartrazine food and medicinal dye, *Med. Nutr.*, 16, 171, 1980.
64. Pellegrin, A., Deux observations nouvelles d'allergie à la tartrazine, *Ann. Med. Interne*, 130, 211, 1979.
65. Miller, K., Sensitivity to tartrazine, *Br. Med. J.*, 285, 1597, 1982.
66. Gangolli, S. D., Grasso, P., Golberg, L., and Hooson, J., Protein binding by food colourings in relation to the production of subcutaneous sarcoma, *Food Cosmet. Toxicol.*, 10, 449, 1972.
67. Jones, R., Ryan, A. J., and Wright, S. E., The metabolism and excretion of tartrazine in the rat, rabbit and man, *Food Cosmet. Toxicol.*, 2, 447, 1964.
68. Walker, R., The metabolism of azo compounds: a review of the literature, *Food Cosmet. Toxicol.*, 8, 659, 1970.
69. Johnson, H. M., Peeler, J. T., and Smith, B. G., Tartrazine: quantitative passive hemagglutination. Studies on a food-borne allergen of small molecular weight, *Immunochemistry*, 8, 281, 1971.
70. Johnson, H. M. and Smith, B. G., Haptenic relationships of p-azobenzenesulphonate and some structurally-related food dyes, *Immunochemistry*, 9, 253, 1972.
71. Nicklin, S. and Miller, K., Induction of a transient reagenic antibody to tartrazine in an animal model, *Int. Arch. Allergy Appl. Immunol.*, 76, 185, 1985.

72. Tada, T., Okumura, K., and Taniguelui, M., Regulation of homocytotoropic antibody formation in the rat, *J. Immunol.*, 141, 952, 1973.
73. Soothill, J. F., Prevention of atropic allergic disease, *Ann. Allergy*, 51, 229, 1983.
74. Kauffman, P. E., Johnson, H. M., and Peeler, J. T., Protein binding of tartrazine and aspirin: an equilibrium study, *IRCS Med. Sci.*, 5, 175, 1977.
75. Weliky, N. and Heiner, D. C., Hypersensitivity to chemicals. Correlation of tartrazine hypersensitivity with characteristic serum IgD and IgE immune response pattern, *Clin. Allergy*, 10, 375, 1980.
76. Bringel, P. J., Vela, C., Urena, V., Gurbindo, D., Garcia, R., and Lahoz, C., IgG antibodies: in vitro blocking activity of IgE mediated reactions, *Clin. Allergy*, 37, 1982.
77. Josephs, S. H. and Buckley, R. H., Serum IgD concentrations in normal infants, children and adults and in patients with elevated IgE, *J. Pediatr.*, 96, 417, 1980.
78. Report, Joint Committee Roy. Coll. Phys. Br. Nutrition Foundation, Food intolerance and food aversion, *J. R. Coll. Physicians London*, 18, 83, 1984.
79. Fisher, A. A., *Contact Dermititis*, Lea & Febiger, Philadelphia, 1973, chap. 2.
80. National Food Institute, Denmark, Rep. No. 43, 1980.
81. Soothill, J. F., Stokes, C. R., Turner, M. W., Norman, A. D., and Taylor, B., Predisposing factors and the development of a reagenic allergy in infancy, *Clin. Allergy*, 6, 305, 1976.
82. Dansset, J. and Svejgaard, A., *HLA and Disease*, Munksgaard, Copenhagen, 1977.
83. Jones, D. H., May, A. G., and Condemi, J. J., HLA DR typing of aspirin sensitive asthmatics, *Ann. Allergy*, 52, 87, 1984.
84. Bodmer, W. F., The HLA system and disease: the Oliver Sharpey Lecture 1979, *J. R. Coll. Physicians London*, 14, 43, 1980.
85. Rosenstreich, D. L., Genetics of resistance to infection, *Nature*, 285, 436, 1980.

Chapter 8

THE INVESTIGATION OF SECRETORY AND SYSTEMIC IMMUNE RESPONSES TO INGESTED MATERIAL IN ANIMAL MODELS

S. J. Challacombe

TABLE OF CONTENTS

I. Introduction 100

II. The Relationship Between the Systemic and Secretory Systems 101
- A. General Considerations 101
- B. Concurrent Activation 101
- C. Possible Mechanisms 102
- D. Possible Biological Relevance 102

III. Mucosal Immune Responses 102
- A. Animal Models 103
- B. Factors Influencing Secretory Responses to Ingested Material 103
  - 1. Antigen Dose 104
    - a. Frequency of Immunization 104
    - b. Nature of Antigen 105
  - 2. Effect of Age 106
  - 3. Immune Status — Effect of Prior Antigen Exposure 107
  - 4. Duration of Secretory Responses 108
  - 5. Cellular Responses 108
  - 6. Damage by Local Application of Antigen 108

IV. Systemic Immune Responses (Oral Tolerance) 109
- A. Immunization vs. Oral Tolerance 109
- B. Oral Tolerance 110
  - 1. Animal Models 111
  - 2. Main Features of Oral Tolerance 111
- C. Factors Influencing Oral Tolerance 112
  - 1. Nature of the Antigen 112
  - 2. Antigen Dose — Frequency of Antigen Exposure 112
  - 3. Immune Status — Effect of Prior Antigen Exposure 113
    - a. Duration of Tolerance 114
  - 4. Genetic Differences 114
  - 5. Gut Flora/LPS 115
  - 6. Antigen-Presenting Cells (APC) 115
- D. Mechanisms of Oral Tolerance 115
  - 1. Cellular Factors 116

V. Relevance of Animal Models to Man 118

VI. Conclusions 119

References 120

I. INTRODUCTION

The use of animal models in the study of immune responses to ingested material has been fundamental to our understanding of many normal aspects of immunology as well as the development of models for diseases of animals and man and also the development of vaccines against human and animal diseases. The success of animal models in enhancing understanding of the immunology of the gastrointestinal tract generally has led to the development of more sophisticated laboratory techniques in an attempt to unravel the complexities of the immune responses and the regulation of these responses. This understanding is a prerequisite of the use of animals as models for diseases of man. The use in the laboratory of many animals where they can be bred under controlled conditions has been particularly important in the study of genetic factors in relation to immune responses and disease.

A variety of animal species including rats, mice, hamsters, pigs, rabbits, sheep, cows, and nonhuman primates have been used in the study of the normal gastrointestinal immune function. In the field of immunology of the gastrointestinal tract, most information has come from experiments in rats and mice. More recently, much information has come from studies using nonhuman primates; this work has been extended to domestic and farm animals. Much of the work in larger animals is based on the investigation of animal diseases and not used as a model for human gastrointestinal responses. Nevertheless, this work has allowed comparisons between species to be made and general conclusions to be drawn. In this review, I shall discuss separately the secretory and systemic immune responses in animal models after ingestion of antigenic material, though for a more detailed account of immunoglobin A (IgA) responses the reader is referred to Chapter 3 (Volume I).

During the last 15 years, significant advances have been made in understanding the intestinal immune system. Much has been learned about the importance of humoral antibody responses at mucosal surfaces and their regulation. Rather less has been learned about the importance of cell-mediated immune responses at mucosal surfaces. There has been extensive characterization of the cells involved and the relationship between antigen-sensitive cells in the intestine and extraintestinal sites.

The intestinal lymphoid cell populations participate in immune responses that are essential components of the host interaction with his environment. Food antigens and bacterial, parasitic, and chemical antigens encountered in the gut present a normal and major antigenic challenge throughout the life of the host. These appeared to be important in the development and function of the host immune system. The mucosal immune system can be regarded as functioning to counteract and handle a major antigenic challenge which is present continually. The nature of these interactions between the host immune system and environmental antigens on mucosal surfaces has been extensively studied and characterized in the last few years.

It is now quite clear that antigen encountered by the enteric route can stimulate antibody responses in the intestine in the absence of any detectable systemic immune responses. Besredka[1] and Davies[2] recognized many years ago that the stools of patients with dysentery may contain a high titer of anti-*Shigella* antibodies, whereas antibodies could not be detected in the serum. It has now been established with a variety of antigens that specific IgA antibody can be induced in the intestine which might mediate local protective immunity.[3-5] The production of secretory antibody may be very localized, and in a number of experiments it has been shown that application of antigen to one segment of the gut may lead to antibodies in that section but not necessarily in others segments.

While it has been demonstrated that antigen given orally may not give rise to serum antibodies, it has also become clear that depending on the conditions used, enteric antigen administration can also result either in enhancement of a systemic immune response[6] or hyporesponsiveness of the systemic immune response.[7,8] The different types of systemic immune responses after oral immunization have now been studied in some detail, using a variety of different antigens, test systems, and animal models. Various types of immune responses have been assessed including antibody-forming cells, humoral antibody, delayed type hypersensitivity, cytotoxic responses, and proliferative responses. With few exceptions it seems that there is some uniformity to conclusions on these experiments, which is that feeding soluble antigens gives rise to antigen-specific systemic hyporesponsiveness. The results in different animal models are discussed in further detail below.

II. THE RELATIONSHIP BETWEEN THE SYSTEMIC AND SECRETORY SYSTEMS

A. General Considerations

It has become clear over the last few years that deposition of antigenic material in the gut may have implications for both the systemic and the mucosal immune systems. Several groups of investigators have examined the systemic responses after such immunization, and the concept of oral tolerance[9] has arisen to describe the phenomenon of specific systemic hyporesponsiveness to soluble antigens which have previously been given by the oral route.[10-16] This was first described in the scientific literature by Wells[7] in 1911, was expanded in the classical experiments of Chase[8] in 1946, and has received thorough analysis in the last few years.[17-20]

At the same time as the latter experiments into systemic hyporesponsiveness were being undertaken, other goups of workers were examining mucosal responses to antigen in the gut. The older concept that antibodies in secretions of the gut and other mucosal surfaces were derived from serum was shown to be incorrect, and it was established on the basis of a variety of criteria that antibodies in secretions were locally derived.[21] Secretory antibodies were mainly of the IgA class; the IgA in secretions were dimeric, whereas serum IgA was monomeric. Antibodies could be induced by local immunization, and antibody levels in secretions did not correlate with those in serum. Early work on the mucosal responses of the gut to antigenic material concentrated almost entirely on analyses of localized responses to antigen, since at that time it had not been appreciated that there might be effects at sites quite distant from the gut.

In recent years it has become apparent that the lymphoid tissue of the gut plays a role in most species which extends far beyond that of the gut, but which is still concerned with the secretory system. The gut-associated lymphoid tissue (GALT) seems to be responsible for the provision of IgA precursor cells not only to the gut but to most other secretory tissues[22] (see Chapter 2 [Volume I]). Thus deposition of antigenic material into the gut may lead to the production of antibodies in the small and large intestines and also in distant secretions such as saliva.[23,24] This system has also received extensive attention in the last few years, though usually by different groups and using different animal models from those groups who have been analyzing oral tolerance.

B. Concurrent Activation

The pertinent question of whether both the secretory system and the induction of oral tolerance can be stimulated by the same immunization schedule and whether the conditions are similar for both has been addressed by a few authors. Swarbrick et al.[25] showed in rats that feeding of antigen leads not only to suppression of the induction of serum antibodies but also to a reduction in the subsequent absorption of antigen in the gut. This was assumed to be a function of local immunity though this was not formally proven. Antigen exclusion after similar immunization schedules has been shown in the elegant experiments of Walker et al.[26] and was shown to be due to secretory IgA (SIgA) antibodies in the small bowel. Challacombe and Tomasi[27] examined the induction of salivary antibodies and systemic tolerance after oral immunization. They showed in mice that prior feeding of ovalbumin led to a dose-dependent suppression of a proliferative response in draining lymph nodes after a subcutaneous challenge. At the higher doses of antigen, salivary antibodies were detected and thus it seemed that in these animals both oral tolerance and salivary IgA antibodies were induced by the same immunization. A single intragastric immunization with 1 mg of ovalbumin led to oral tolerance but did not lead to detectable SIgA antibodies, whereas 10 mg of ovalbumin led to oral tolerance and salivary IgA antibodies.

C. Possible Mechanisms

A possible explanation of how immunity and tolerance can be induced concurrently is that suppressor, helper, and antibody precursor cells are all induced in Peyer's patches by oral immuniztion. Richman et al.[28] in in vitro systems have been able to show that oral immunization leads to the induction in Peyer's patches of suppressor cells for IgG and helper cells for IgA responses. An extension of this idea to in vivo conditions would suggest that the suppression of systemic serum IgG responses might be due to suppressor cells, whereas helper cells for IgA may explain the SIgA responses, particularly if these were to migrate to secretory tissues. However, in other work discussed in more detail below, it has been reported that serum IgG, IgA, and IgM antibody responses might be suppressed at the same time as salivary IgA antibodies are present. This would indicate that suppressor cells are present for systemic IgA responses and that SIgA responses escape this suppression perhaps due to helper cells which are specific for secretory sites. There is some evidence of homing of both T and B cells to secretory tissues as discussed below.

D. Possible Biological Relevance

In man, an inverse relationship between serum IgG and salivary IgA antibodies has also been reported with antibody directed to *Streptococcus mutans*.[29] Sequential studies indicated that as serum IgG antibodies increased in response to the development of dental caries, salivary IgA antibodies decreased. Conversely, when serum IgG antibodies decreased, salivary IgA antibodies were found to increase.[29] These observations indicate some active relationship between the two systems. The demonstration of this relationship and the observation that intragastric immunization may lead to simultaneous induction of secretory antibodies and systemic suppression raises intriguing speculation as to the relationship between the two systems and the biological relevance of these observations. The occurrence of a secretory immune response after mucosal contact with antigen would appear to be a most useful mechanism with regard to the exclusion of potentially harmful substances from the body.[26] The induction of systemic tolerance could act as a secondary defense to ensure that immunologically damaging reactions to antigens that escape exclusion do not occur. This may be a particularly appropriate response with regard to various allergens[11,13] which might otherwise have harmful effects on the body. It may also be an appropriate response to antigens that cross-react with self and therefore might induce autoimmunity; this is an area which deserves further attention.

III. MUCOSAL IMMUNE RESPONSES

The development of immunocompetency in mammals occurs during fetal life.[30,31] The lymphatic tissue of the intestine reacts to antigenic stimulae by rapid development which is particularly apparent during the first days after birth.[32] It has become evident that the gut is closely associated with other mucosal surfaces and that IgA precursor cells originate in Peyer's patches and are stimulated by intestinal antigens to leave the Peyer's patch, migrate through the mesenteric lymph nodes (MLN), the thoracic duct, and blood, and return to the gut and a variety of other mucosal surfaces. This has been described as the common mcusoal system.[33,34] A similar pathway appears to be true for T cells originating in the gut, and these also migrate to other mucosal surfaces.[35] Thus the gastrointestinal tract appears to be intimately associated with other mucosal surfaces.

The deposition of antigens in the gut has been shown to lead to the production of IgA antibodies in secretions at sites distant from the gut such as colostrum, lacrimal and salivary secretions in man[23] and salivary secretions in rhesus monkeys[24] and in rats.[36] A general conclusion therefore is that the secretory immune system can be stimulated centrally and that percursors of IgA-producing cells migrate from the GALT to several secretory sites in addition to the lamina propria of the gut itself.

A. Animal Models

Several species have secretory systems analagous to that described in man. These include the monkey, rabbit, dog, guinea pig, rat, mouse, hamster, cat, and hedgehog.[37] In these species, IgA is the predominant Ig in secretions including saliva and milk. In most of these species, the physicochemical properties of the predominant form of IgA in secretions is similar to that of man with a sedimentation coefficient of about 11S. In the monkey, dog, cow, rabbit, and guinea pig a polypeptide chain probably similar to the secretory component (SC) has been detected.[21] There appears to be antigenic cross-reactivity between the SC of man, monkey, and cow, and the IgA of other species such as the chicken, dolphin, and seal will combine with human SC.[21]

These various species have secretory systems which appear to be analagous to that described in man on the basis of immunochemical studies. However, in several of these species the mechanisms involved in the actual induction of secretory antibodies has not been examined, particularly with regard to the stimulation of secretory responses by intragastric or intraduodenal immunization. In addition, there are quantitative differences between the species with regard to the IgG content of secretions such as saliva. For example in the rat, almost 50% of the total Ig in saliva appears to be IgG,[38] whereas in primates, IgG only accounts for about 2% of the total Ig.[39]

Salivary antibody induction has been widely used as a model system to analyze secretory responses to ingested material, primarily because saliva is an easy secretion to collect and analyze. It seems to be a general feature that salivary IgA antibodies can be induced in a variety of species in the absence of serum antibodies (Table 1). This has been demonstrated after immunization with particulate bacterial antigens in humans,[23] monkeys,[24] rabbits,[40] rats,[36] and mice.[27] The appearance of salivary antibodies after immunization or intragastric deposition of soluble antigens has been less widely reported, though salivary antibodies after intragastric immunization with BGG (bovine gammaglobulin) has been reported in rabbits by Montgomery et al.[40] and in mice using ovalbumin[27] and antigen I/II, a soluble protein antigen derived from *S. mutans*.[6]

The local production of antibodies will not be discussed further, though it should be borne in mind that most secretions can be stimulated either locally or centrally and that many studies have shown that local antibody responses are best stimulated by local application of antigen. The induction of IgA antibodies is discussed in detail in Chapter 2 (Volume I).

B. Factors Influencing Secretory Responses to Ingested Material

The main secretions which have been examined with regard to the induction of se-

Table 1
FACTORS WHICH HAVE BEEN SHOWN TO INFLUENCE THE INDUCTION OF SECRETORY ANTIBODY OR SYSTEMIC TOLERANCE BY INGESTION OF ANTIGEN

Frequency of immunization (exposure)
Dosage of antigen
Nature of antigen
Soluble or particulate
Viable or nonviable (vaccines)
Age of animals
Species of animal
Prior exposure — immune status of animal
APC
Site of immunization

cretory responses after materials have been ingested have been those in the gut and in saliva. Saliva has been selected not only because of its relevance in oral disease but mainly because it is an accessible fluid, easy to collect, and thought to be representative of responses in secretions after central or intragastric immunization. There are a number of factors which influence successful induction of secretory antibody by this route (Table 1).

1. Antigen Dose

It has been a general finding from many studies in a variety of species that very large antigen doses are needed to induce a secretory response after deposition of antigen in the gut. Thus in mice, Michalek et al.[36] delivered 10^{10} bacteria daily for 10 days to get a salivary response, while in pigs, Dziaba et al.[41] gave greater than 10^{11} and in man, Dupont et al.[42] found that 10^{12} was optimal. Interestingly, in the experiments involved with vaccination against disease, the protection achieved was incomplete and usually inferior to natural infection or vaccination with living organisms. Several studies have analyzed dose responses with regard to the secretory system. The results suggest that there may be a window of responsiveness in a wall of unresponsiveness. In the studies of Michalek et al.[36] and Challacombe,[6] nonresponsiveness was found in the lowest and highest of three immunization doses. Thus giving mice either 5×10^8 or 5×10^{10} organisms on three consecutive days did not result in a detectable salivary antibody response. However, salivary antibody titers were detected[6] after administration of 5×10^9. The fact that in both these studies there was an upper limit of responsiveness suggests that the secretory system can be hyporesponsive if the antigen dose is large enough.

a. Frequency of Immunization

The frequency of immunization is another factor which has been considered. In experiments in man, 12 daily intragastric immunizations with *S. mutans* resulted in successful induction of secretory antibodies in parotid and submandibular saliva and the lacrimal secretions.[23] A similar regime resulted in antibodies in secretion in monkeys,[24] though failures have also been reported using similar regimes in the monkey model.[43,44] In rats, Taubman and Smith[45] have orally immunized up to 24 times to induce salivary antibodies. However, schedules of less frequent immunization were not examined. We have examined the minimum immunization schedule which would give rise to salivary antibody responses after oral immunization. Although a single immunization can sometimes give rise to detectable antibody responses, a more consistent response is found with a minimum of three or four oral immunizations.[6] In contrast, weekly immunizations over several months did not give rise to a consistent response to saliva. Thus not only the antigen dose but also the frequency of immunization seems to be critical in inducing secretory antibody responses.

b. Nature of Antigen

It is a general finding that living organisms orally administered appeared to have greater immunogenicity than inactivated oral vaccines. The greater response and functional capacity in terms of protection elicited by viable organisms has been reported by a large number of workers who have used a variety of organisms including *Vibrio cholera, Escherichia coli, Salmonella typhimurium,* and *Shigella.*[4,46-48] It seems possible that in order to elicit a strong response that colonization of the intestinal tract with the immunizing strain is necessary. This is supported by some work with poliovirus and by observations that in experiments in pigs with *E. coli* that local antibody production was detected only in animals in which the organisms could be cultured from the feces.[49] Interestingly, animals lacking a binding receptor for the K88 antigen of *E. coli,* which is involved in adherence, did not give a satisfactory response to the *E. coli.*[50]

Thus in the field of oral vaccines, attention has recently turned to immunization with attenuated strains which might colonize the gut such as nonpathogenic strains of *Salmonella typhimurium* which have been used in cows.[47] This approach has been extended to humans and the interesting work with the attenuated strain of *S. typhimurium* substrain Ty21a which lacks an enzyme essential to the utilization of galactose which limits its survival in the host has been most promising, and it seems also to produce effective protection in man.[51,52]

However, in terms of safety there are obvious advantages in using inactivated oral vaccines, and this is the most straightforward and obvious method of oral immunization. In general, the results of feeding inactivated whole organisms on the induction of secretory responses have been much more capricious than using live vaccines. The doses of antigen needed to induce any secretory response (see below) have been very large, and with whole bacteria range from 10^{10} organisms in mice[36] to 10^{11} and 10^{12} in calves[53] and in man.[41]

The larger doses needed may reflect the relative inefficiency of sampling in the gastrointestinal tract; it may indicate that as discussed above, organisms need to adhere to the mucosa to be effective immunogens; and it may reflect that the antigen is greatly diluted in the environment of the gut. The implications of these findings with regard to responses to ingested material are that it would seem that either large doses of antigen or frequent exposure to antigen is needed to have a detectable response in secretions distant from the gut.

As the results in Table 2 indicate, in general, particulate antigens have been rather more effective, whether viable or inactivated, in inducing secretory antibodies than have soluble antigens. This particular aspect has been examined in more detail recently.[6,54] A comparison of salivary antibody responses after oral immunization in mice of ovalbumin and inactivated *Streptococcus mutans* indicated that the responses with the streptococcus were always greater. In addition an anamnestic response could be induced with whole cells of *S. mutans* but not with ovalbumin. This result was confirmed in subsequent experiments comparing soluble antigen with that insolubilized on Sepharose® beads. The antigen used as a soluble protein of 185,000 mol wt was derived from *S. mutans.* As seen in Figure 1, when antigen was given intragastrically on three occasions into mice in the soluble or insoluble form, a similar response was detected in saliva. However, when animals were given a second series of immunizations

Table 2
INDUCTION OF SALIVARY ANTIBODIES BY STIMULATION OF GALT

Species	Antigen	Route	Salivary IgA Abs	Serum Abs	Ref.
Human	*Streptococcus mutans*	Oral	++	−	23
Monkeys	*S. mutans*	Intragastric	++	−	24
Rabbits	Pneumococcus/BGG	Intragastric	++	−	40
Rats	*S. mutans*	Oral	++	−	36
Mice	*S. mutans*/ovalbumin	Intragastric	++	−	27

Note: Serum antibodies are not induced normally in unprimed animals.

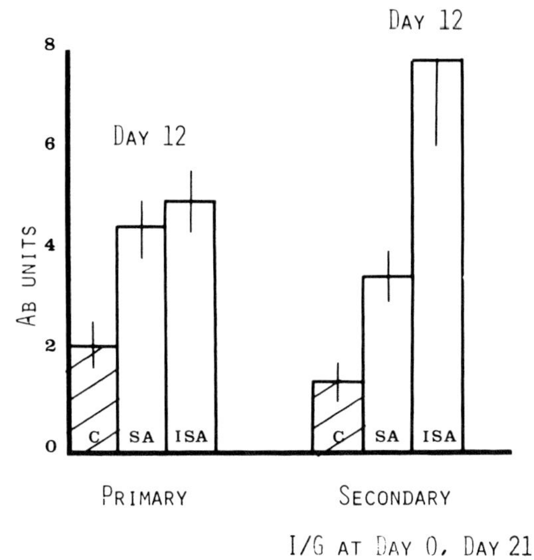

FIGURE 1. Salivary antibodies after intragastric immunization of BALB/c mice with soluble (SA) or insoluble (ISA) streptococcal antigen. Groups of six mice were given three daily immunizations of 50 μg of antigen on days 0, 1, and 2 and a second series on days 21, 22, and 33. Salivary antibody titers are shown for days 12 and day 33 (12 days after second series).

intragastrically some weeks later, the antigen in the insoluble form gave a significantly greater response than in the soluble form. This can be interpreted as evidence of an anamnestic response in secretions though not classical of those described with systemic responses. The nature of antigens also has implications with regard to the systemic immune responses (see below), since in general soluble antigens give rise to oral tolerance, while particulate antigens do not.

2. Effect of Age

There has been relatively little work in animal models on the effects of age on secretory antibody responses. In man the secretory system is thought to mature in advance of the systemic immune system in terms of IgA. Recent work suggests that the IgA levels in whole unstimulated saliva, which may be representative of the mucosal immune system, reach adult values at between 1 and 2 years of age.[55] It had been assumed previously that the SIgA system matured even faster.[56] It is not known whether the

Table 3
THE EFFECT OF AGE ON THE INDUCTION OF SALIVARY ANTIBODIES TO *STREPTOCOCCUS MUTANS* BY INTRAGASTRIC IMMUNIZATION

Age (weeks)	Control	Immunized
5	2.1 ± 0.3	0.5 ± 0.2
11	0.6 ± 0.5	2.8 ± 0.3[a]
17	1.3 ± 0.5	5.7 ± 0.5[a]
52	1.8 ± 0.4	2.1 ± 0.7

Note: CBA/CA mice given 10^{10} *S. mutans* intragastrically on 3 consecutive days, saliva assayed 14 days later, results expressed as mean antibody units mℓ ± SE of groups of six mice.

[a] $p<0.01$.

IgA response shows any decrease in old age. In mice, the salivary IgA response does appear to be age dependent. The salivary response to either soluble protein antigens or to whole bacteria was greater in mature animals of 17 weeks of age or greater than in young animals. Since no differences were found in the systemic IgA antibody responses in young or mature mice, it is possible that maturation of the secretory system is delayed in comparison with the immune system in mice, even though this is the reverse of that found in man. In these experiments (Table 3), it was not possible to induce responses in aged animals, and it is therefore possible that the secretory immune system becomes less efficient with age. However, further work is needed in this area and in other animal models.

3. *Immune Status — Effect of Prior Antigen Exposure*

In some studies it has been possible to stimulate the production of mucosal antibody by nonmucosal presentation of antigen. Svennerholm et al.[57] showed that a subcutaneous vaccination with *Vibrio cholera* could induce immunity in secretions of women who had been previously sensitized to cholera. Other studies have examined the concept of systemic priming with oral boosting, and Pierce and Gowans[58] found that with cholera toxin a single intraperitoneal injection in adjuvant followed 2 weeks later with intestinal immunization produced a maximal IgA antitoxin response which peaked 4 days after the boost. This regime was shown by the same authors to be protective in the dog. Protection of lambs from *Salmonella typhimurium* infection has been shown also to be effectively induced by a combination of systemic priming and oral boost.[59]

This would seem to suggest that secretory responses are enhanced by prior systemic sensitization. Unfortunately, this combination does not seem to be universal and in other experiments, subcutaneous priming of rabbits followed by oral dosing has been shown to suppress subsequent IgA antibody responses.[60] Similar results have been shown with sheep.[61] Thus it seems that the animal species and the nature of the antigen are as important as whether the animals have had prior systemic exposure to the antigen.

With regard to previous exposure of the secretory system alone or previous antigen exposure in the gut, the results from different animal models vary with respect to the evidence for immunological memory within the secretory immune system. As discussed earlier, oral immunization in man leads to a modified secondary response in secretions which is larger than but of similar duration to the primary response.[23] In monkeys, a secondary series of intragastric immunizations gave rise to a similar response with no evidence of an anamnestic response.[24] It has been shown that orally immunized rabbits may show an anamnestic response in the mammary gland,[62] and rats immunized by injection into the Peyer's patches with suboptimal doses of antigen produce a more rapid and greater biliary IgA response on challenge up to a year later.[63] Taken overall, the results suggest that the nature of the secretory response to ingested material may certainly depend on prior antigen exposure but that this may vary according to the nature of the antigen.

4. Duration of Secretory Responses

It has been a general finding from animal models that the duration of secretory responses after gut immunization is short lived. In experiments reported in mice,[6,64] secretory responses have been detectable 1 to 2 weeks after immunization but diminished by 3 or 4 weeks. In man, the secretory antibody responses in lacrimal and salivary secretions after intragastric immunization with *Streptococcus mutans* lasted for a total of approximately 6 weeks.[23] A secondary immunization gave antibodies of a similar duration, though these appeared to give a modified type of secondary response in that the titers were larger. Similar short-lived responses have been found in monkeys,[24] and in rabbits, secretory responses to the cholera toxin were short lived after intragastric immunization.[59]

These results taken together suggest that after the migration of antigen-sensitive cells of Peyer's patches to secretory tissues the cells do not continue to secrete antibodies in the absence of any local or continued antigenic challenge. Amplification of the local antibody response can be induced if antigen is then applied at individual sites.[65]

5. Cellular Responses

It is clear that cell-mediated mechanisms may be activated by antigenic material in the gut. Cells capable of responding to and stimulating mixed lymphocyte reactions have been shown in the lamina propria of the small intestine.[66,67] Feeding of H-2 incompatible cells to mice may lead to the induction of cytotoxic T cells in Peyer's patches and the spleen.[68] Local cell-mediated immunity has also been shown in response to various parasites in rats,[69] mice,[70] and chickens.[71]

The nature of the intraepithelial lymphocyte has been extensively investigated in recent years,[72] and lymphocytes with killer cell or natural killer cell activity have been detected.[73] Experimental models of graft vs. host disease certainly demonstrated the presence of local cell-mediated immunity.[74,75] The normal bacterial flora in mice have been shown to be an important prerequisite for the capability of mediating a delayed hypersensitivity response to ingested antigen.[76] However, it is not known whether this is a general phenomenon, and further work in this area is needed.

6. Damage by Local Application of Antigen

Direct application of antigen to the intestinal mucosa may lead to tissue damage and infiltration of polymorphonuclear leukocytes. In pigs it has been demonstrated by Bellamy and Nielsen[77] that exposure of the mucosa to bovine serum albumin led to the migration of neutrophils into the lumen but that this was not accompanied by detectable edema or hemorrhage. This reaction was seen within 4 hours of application of antigen. It was postulated that this was a method by which local immunity might be enhanced by neutrophils, but it is clearly a mechanism by which antigens in the gut may cause damage to the mucosa.

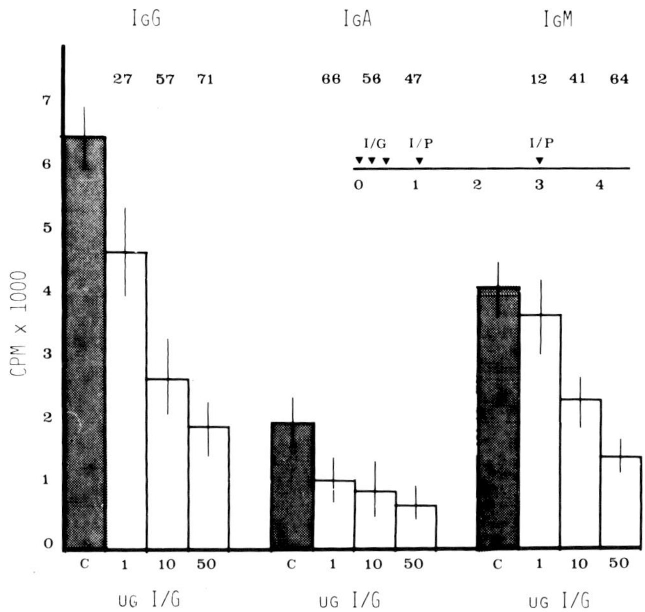

FIGURE 2. Serum antibodies to streptococcal antigen I/II after intragastric (I/G) immunization with soluble antigen and systemic challenge. Mice were given three intragastric doses of Sa I/II followed by intraperitoneal (I/P) challenge with 2 μ of SA I/II in adjuvant 1 and 3 weeks later. Antibodies assayed by solid phase radioassay.

IV. SYSTEMIC IMMUNE RESPONSES (ORAL TOLERANCE)

A. Immunization vs. Oral Tolerance

Deposition of antigen in the gut may lead either to immunization in the systemic immune system (enhancement) or to hyporesponsiveness (oral tolerance). Whether priming or tolerance occurs is dependent on a number of complex immunoregulatory mechanisms, the nature of the antigen, and whether the animals had prior exposure to the antigen. Although presentation of antigen by the enteric route appears to prime particularly well for local immune responses of the IgA class,[78] this is not exclusive to this isotype.[79]

In the dog, Pierce and Costa[80] have shown that if animals are given cholera toxoid intraperitoneally in adjuvant 2 weeks before oral immunization of cholera toxin, then this leads to an enhanced mucosal anticholera response and also an augmented systemic response. In studies with mice, we have been able to show that oral immunization with ovalbumin leads to systemic hyporesponsiveness; however, if the animals have been primed, then the same immunization may give rise to enhanced systemic IgG antibody responses. This concept has important implications as to the responses to ingested material, but it is unclear whether this is dependent on the nature of the antigen and whether this applies to both the humoral and the cellular arms of the immune response. The importance of the nature of the antigen is discussed in more detail below.

In experiments comparing soluble with insoluble antigen on the humoral antibody responses in serum and secretions after intragastric immunization with streptococcal antigen I/II, different responses were found according to whether the antigen was soluble (Figure 2) or insoluble (Figure 3). As seen in Figure 3, administration of insoluble streptococcal antigen intragastrically led to a dose-dependent enhancement of the

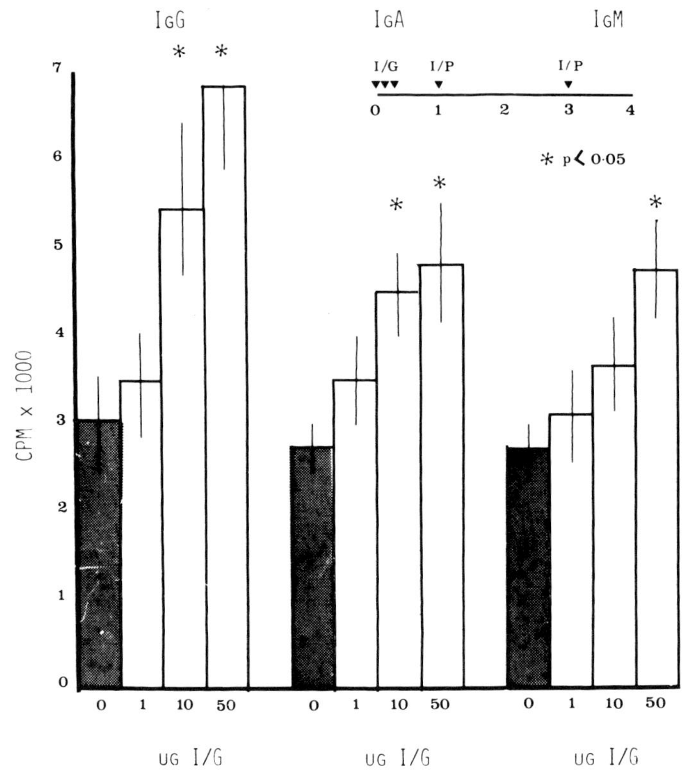

FIGURE 3. Serum antibodies to streptococcal antigen I/II after intragastric immunization with insolubilized SA I/II. Immunization schedule is as indicated in legend for Figure 1.

subsequent systemic immune response of the IgG, IgA, and IgM isotypes. This is similar to that previously described with whole bacteria of *S. mutans.*[6] Serum antibody to the O antigen of *E. coli* was found to be enhanced after feeding *E. coli* to pigs.[81] Similarly, mice fed *E. coli* showed an increased serum antibody response to the somatic antigen.[82] With bacterial antigens, it is unclear whether the enhanced systemic response is due to the nature of the antigen itself or to prior exposure to similar or cross-reacting antigens. In the example shown in Figure 3 with insolubilized streptococcal antigen, it seemed unlikely that prior exposure was the explanation, since giving the same antigen in the soluble form resulted in dose-dependent suppression of the systemic humoral antibody response[54] (see Figure 2.) Thus it seems that the nature of the antigen itself is one of the most important influences on whether systemic tolerance or enhancement occurs after the ingestion of antigen.

B. Oral Tolerance

It has been known since the work of Besredka[83] in 1909 and Wells[7] in 1911 that animals fed soluble proteins lose their ability to respond to this specific antigen on subsequent systemic challenge. More recently, many investigators have studied the systemic hyporesponsiveness after enteric antigen administration. While in certain situations this type of immunization can result in priming (see below), there is an impressive degree of agreement that despite marked differences in experimental design such as feeding protocols, species of the experimental animals used, and the type of response measured, the ingestion of antigen will lead to systemic hyporesponisveness. A common feature of all these studies has been the fact that the immunological unresponsive-

Table 4
SOME EXAMPLES OF ORAL TOLERANCE

Species	Antigens	Route	Assay	Ref
Guinea pig	Ovalbumin	Oral	PCA	7
	DNCB	Oral	DTH	8
Mice	SRBC	Intragastric	PFC	10
	Ovalbumin	Intragastric	PCA	11
	Ovalbumin	Intragastric	PA	16
	Picryl chloride	Oral	DTH	12
	Antigen I/II	Intragastric	Antibody	6
Rats	SRBC	Oral	PFC	15
Pigs	BGG	Oral	Antibody	49

ness after such antigen feeding is to a remarkable degree antigen specific. Hyporesponsiveness has been shown in both humoral and cellular arms of the systemic response.

1. Animal Models

A variety of animal models have been used in the study or oral tolerance. An impressive degree of concordance throughout the various experiments indicates that this is a response which may have wide biological relevance and certainly is present with regard to the response to food antigens in man. Some examples of animal models are shown in Table 4. The guinea pig was the first animal model to be examined scientifically in this system, and both Wells[7] and Chase[8] used this animal model to show depressed passive cutaneous anaphylaxis (PCA) and delayed hypersensitivity (DTH), respectively, after feeding of antigen or hapten. However, most investigators have used either mice or rats in attempts to understand and dissect some of the mechanisms underlying this phenomenon. Thus in mice, the various authors have assayed PCA, DTH, and plaque-forming cells (PFC). Proliferative assays have been used to determine T cell responses,[16,27] and serum antibody has been measured by others.[18,25,84] Few larger animals have been used, though diminished serum responses in pigs have been reported.[85] Some evidence exists in man that ingestion of antigenic material may result in systemic hyporesponsiveness.[86] There is some debate as to the exact mechanisms involved in the induction of oral tolerance in each of the different systems, and this is discussed in more detail below.

2. Main Features of Oral Tolerance

As evidenced in Table 4, oral tolerance can affect different aspects of the immune response. Hyporesponsiveness of systemic antibody reduction has been manifested by the demonstration that serum antibody levels of all three isotypes can be reduced.[6] Many authors have examined PFC and have shown that animals given oral antigen have reduced numbers of splenic IgM and IgG PFC though few authors have examined IgA.[10,14] The demonstration that systemic antibodies and PCA can be inhibited in orally immunized animals[13,87] suggests that IgE responses are also depressed. In fact suppressor cells for IgE have been shown in Peyer's patches.[13]

Orally induced tolerance can certainly affect cell-mediated responses, and several authors have examined DTH reactions after such oral immunization.[12,20,88] The proliferation of antigen-stimulated lymphocytes in vitro is also reduced in animals given oral antigen.[27] A striking feature of oral tolerance is the degree of specificity. This applies to both the humoral and cellular arms of the systemic immune response. Thus many authors have shown that being fed ovalbumin tolerizes animals to this protein but not to unrelated antigens such as human γ-globulin (HGG) and human serum albumin.[18,27,88]

It should be noted that oral tolerance applies primarily to T cell-dependent antigens and that the tolerance is maintained at the T cell level. It seems likely that in most instances the B cell itself is not tolerized.[21] While tolerance is a very common feature in animal models following ingestion of antigenic material, this is not an absolutely consistent response. A number of factors will determine whether tolerance or immunization results as discussed above, and one of the most important of these appears to be the immune status of the animal. Thus it is difficult to detect the tolerizing effects of intragastric immunization or feeding in animals which already have been primed systemically, and this will be discussed further. There is also some evidence of species differences with regard to systemic responses to orally administered protein antigens, and there are also detectable genetic differences (see below).

C. Factors Influencing Oral Tolerance

1. Nature of the Antigen

The tolerogenicity of an orally delivered antigen is determined by a number of factors including its degree of T dependance but also by other properties such as whether it is particulate or soluble, easily digested by proteases or resistant, or easily aggregated or survives in the intestinal tract. There are differences between antigens in their ability to induce oral tolerance, which may depend on their mechanical structure. For example, soluble proteins can lead to a long-lasting systemic tolerance (and an active mucosal response), whereas tolerance to more complex antigens such as cell walls of bacteria may require larger amounts of antigen for tolerance induction and this tolerance may be relatively short lived.[27,89] With certain complex antigens such as *S. mutans,* a significant proliferative response may be found in Peyer's patches within the 10 days following feeding, whereas no proliferate response was detected with soluble proteins such as ovalbumin or KLH.[27]

The importance of the role of the antigen structure is demonstrated by studies with cholera,[89] where it seems that antigen combinations may be more effective than antigens given singly. Analysis of the mechanisms of oral tolerance after antigen feeding is made more challenging by the observation that with certain complex antigens like bacteria, oral tolerance may be seen to one of the surface antigens and yet enhancement to another.[82] This presumably may be due to prior exposure to antigens which cross-react with one but not another of the surface antigens.

Although most studies have been performed with protein antigens, it has been demonstrated that humoral antibody responses to the polysaccharide dextran B 1355 can be markedly diminished following oral feeding. Thus Kagnoff[90] showed that the IgM and IgA PFC responses in spleens were markedly diminished following feeding. The B 1355 is thought to be a thymus-independent antigen. In contrast, Chiller et al.[91] found that feeding lipopolysaccaride (LPS), polyvinyl pyrolidone, or TNP-Ficoll did not suppress antibody responses when animals were subsequently challenged with the same antigen. It is possible though that these variances in results may reflect differences in the protocols rather than the effect of the different antigens, since the dextran was fed daily for 6 days (10 mg per dose) before suppression was noted, whereas the other antigens were fed as single doses of 20 mg or as 20 mg divided over 3 days.

The ability of skin-sensitizing agents and haptens to induce oral tolerance has been noted above and indeed is one of the best-analyzed systems following the work of Chase.[8] In a hapten carrier system, the tolerance induced is carrier specific.[92] In other words, it requires challenge with the same carrier and hapten to demonstrate the oral tolerance.

2. Antigen Dose — Frequency of Antigen Exposure

The dosage of antigen and the schedule of feeding seem to be important parameters

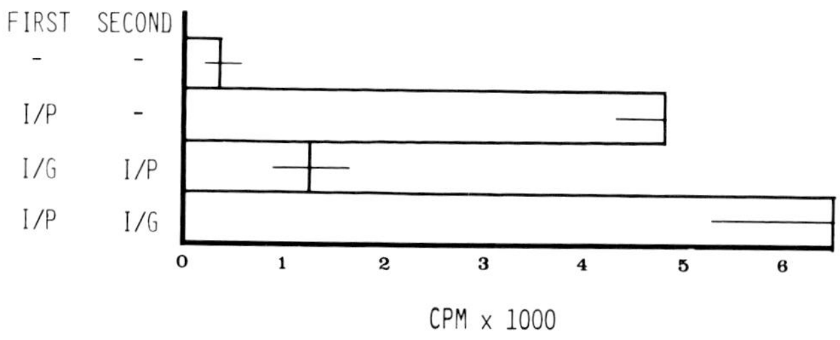

FIGURE 4. Effects of sequence of immunization in subsequent serum IgG antibody response to ovalbumin. Animals were given three daily intragastric (I/G) administrations of ovalbumin (10 mg). Intraperitoneal (I/P) immunization were with 100 μg of ovalbumin in adjuvant. Serum antibodies were assayed by radioimmunoassay.

in the induction of oral tolerance. It is dependent on both the antigen and the animal species examined. For example, with certain contact-sensitizing agents (e.g., oxazolone) small doses such as 0.1 to 1 mg given intragastrically will tolerize the animal, whereas higher doses (10 mg) will lead to sensitization.[93] With a well-studied antigen such as ovalbumin, varying responses have been reported according to antigen dose. Thus oral tolerance to ovalbumin could be achieved by feeding either very small or large doses. It has been reported that with small doses, DTH and IgE antibody formation might be diminished, but higher doses of antigen were required for inhibition of IgG responses.[94,95]

In contrast, it has been reported that feeding of ovalbumin in very small amounts in mice (1 to 100 μg) may prime rather than tolerize animals.[96] In our own experiments in mice with ovalbumin, we have found a wide range of antigen doses capable of inducing oral tolerance. Thus with cell-mediated responses, single oral doses of between 1 and 20 mg gave rise to oral tolerance,[27] and a similar range of antigen doses gave rise to suppression of the humoral antibody response in terms of the IgG, IgA, and IgM isotypes.[6] This wide range of antigen doses giving rise to oral tolerance is in contrast to the narrow range of antigen doses which can give rise to the induction of secretory IgA antibodies.

3. Immune Status — Effect of Prior Antigen Exposure

The immune status of the animal appears to be a critical determinant with respect to the type of systemic response to ingested antigen. Thus in mice it has been demonstrated that soluble antigen given to an immunologically virgin animal may result in oral tolerance, whereas if the same amount of antigen is given to a primed animal, enhancement of the subsequent systemic response may be seen.[54] An example is shown in Figure 4, where a comparison was made of the effect of the sequence of immunization on the serum IgG antibodies to ovalbumin. If an intraperitoneal immunization was preceded by intragastric immunization, tolerance occurred. However, if the intraperitoneal immunization was followed by an intragastric immunization, the IgG antibody response was greater than with the intraperitoneal immunization alone.

These observations suggest that prior sensitization may have profound effects on the nature of the systemic response and raises the question of which conditions might allow feeding of antigen to tolerize an already primed host. Recent studies[97] suggest that in mice, subsequent feeding abrogates the serum antibody response of parenterally immunized mice. Partial systemic tolerance has been reported in primed rats after prolonged oral administration of antigen.[98] This, however, is not a universal finding, and it is a most important point in terms of the potential of treatment by the oral route of previously sensitized patients. Thus more work is needed in this area to determine the exact parameters which might result in enhancement or tolerance in already primed subjects.

One of these parameters seems to be prolonged antigen feeding. For example, Kagnoff[14] showed that while short-term feeding of sheep red blood cells (SRBC) boosted the IgA and IgG serum antibody titers in mice, if antigen feeding was continued over longer periods, the animals were tolerized. In a similar system, oral tolerance to SRBC was induced in primed mice by prolonged feeding.[99] This rationale has already been applied in humans in attempts to tolerize allergic patients by oral immunization.[100,101]

Prior passive immuniztion with specific antibodies may reduce the tolerogenic activity of fed ovalbumin.[18] It is not clear whether this can be explained by the antigen being absorbed or bound by circulating antibodies or how this affects the induction of suppressor cells in the Peyer's patch but is an observation which may have biological relevance.

a. Duration of Tolerance

Oral tolerance to most protein antigens and to erythrocytes has been shown to be long lasting in most animal models and in the mice and rats persists for several months.[14,27,102] However, this observation is not universal to all antigens, and in a system in mice where tolerance was induced to *S. mutans*, the tolerance lasted for relatively brief periods.[27] Since in most systems oral tolerance applies primarily to T cell-dependent antigens and the B cell is not tolerized, it is possible that active suppression may be present for much longer periods of time than the adoptive transfer studies have indicated. For example, suppressive factors have been found in extracts of spleen taken from HGG-tolerant animals as long as 4 months after induction of oral tolerance, whereas T suppressor (T_s) cells could only be demonstrated for 3 months.[102] This raises the possibility that relatively low levels of suppressor activity are necessary to maintain T cell unresponsiveness late in tolerance. The mechanisms involved in tolerance are discussed in more detail below.

4. Genetic Differences

As discussed in earlier sections, species differences may be important in the systemic responses to ingested antigen. Decreased DTH responses and decreased antibody responses to parenteral challenge have been reported not only in the various animal models but in humans after mucosal exposure to reactive chemicals or protein antigens.[86,103] However, while results in human models seem to follow the results of most animal models, not all animals response in the same way. For example, feeding of antigens such as bovine serum albumin tolerizes both mice and rats,[84,104] but the same antigen given to rabbits seems to have a priming effect.[105]

Initial studies have shown that oral tolerance may be different from systemic tolerance with regard to genetic control.[102] It seems that within strains bearing the same $H\text{-}2^k$ histocompatibility locus, there are significant differences in the ease of induction of oral tolerance to deaggregated human γ-globulin. This suggests that non-H-2-linked genes are also important in oral tolerance. This would be similar to findings with systemic tolerance where Ranges and Azar[106] have shown that both H-2 and non-H-2 genes influence systemic tolerance. Stokes et al.[107] examined genetic differences in tolerance and the ability to exclude ingested antigen in different strains of mice. Distinct differences were found in the capacity to absorb antigen between the four strains of mice examined, and also differences were detected in the ability to develop oral tolerance.

Taken together, these results clearly suggest that genetic differences exist in the handling of antigen by the gut and are of obvious relevance in man with regard to differential susceptibility to food allergy. It was interesting to note that the ability to develop tolerance did not correlate with the ability to develop immune exclusion, and this suggests that these two functions are inherited independently.[107]

5. Gut Flora/LPS

A number of substances within the lumen may have an effect on the response to a particular antigen. It is known that the normal gut flora has a pronounced effect upon the immune system, and a wide range of immune activities are modified including the ability to mount DTH reactions[76] and macrophage function.[108] Using the mouse model, McGhee et al.[109] have shown that bacterial LPS can profoundly influence the regulation of IgA responses and the generation of tolerance. Feeding with LPS enhances oral tolerance to antigens such as SRBC given at the same time. Thus oral tolerance to SRBC could not be induced in LPS-nonresponsive nor germ-free mice, while in genetically related LPS-responsive and germ-free mice pretreated with LPS, tolerance to SRBC could be induced.[99]

It is possible that LPS derived from the normal microflora contributes to expansion of suppressor cells in the GALT. In the DTH model in mice, feeding of LPS has been shown to enhance oral tolerance to oxazolone and picrylchloride.[110] However, this might not apply to all antigens, since oral tolerance to ovalbumin was induced equally well in LPS-responsive and LPS-nonresponsive mice.[111] It also seems that oral tolerance to an antigen can be avoided if it is given within 48 hr of primary contact with an unrelated antigen.[107] This suggests that a response to an ingested antigen may be modified if an immune response is already being generated to an unrelated antigen. This is clearly an interesting area which deserves further investigation.

6. Antigen-Presenting Cells (APC)

Another factor which may affect either immune regulation or tolerance is the nature of the APC. It has not been excluded that antigen presentation for the induction of IgA-producing cells is mediated by different cells from those for the systemic immune responses. It is also possible that different structural forms of antigen might be handled differentially and account for differences in responses to ingestion of soluble or particulate antigens. Peyer's patches certainly contain cells capable of presenting antigen to induce immune responses. Both macrophages and Ia-positive cells have been found within Peyer's patches.[112]

In addition, Peyer's patch macrophages have been shown to be capable of supporting the induction of immune responses in vitro.[113] However, these functional cells may not be identical to APC elsewhere, since adherent Ia-positive cells from Peyer's patches do not seem to be so effective in antigen presentation.[102,112] The absolute requirement of Peyer's patches and other GALT for the induction of human secretory immunity and oral tolerance has been the subject of much investigation. This will not be reviewed here; while early studies indicated that Peyer's patches were essential, more recent studies have suggested that in addition to the special epithelium of Peyer's patches and lymphoid follicles, other areas of the intestines may be engaged in antigen presentation.[114]

D. Mechanisms of Oral Tolerance

As can be seen from Table 5, in the various animal models a large number of mechanisms have been postulated as underlying oral tolerance. They can be broadly divided into humoral or cellular mechanisms, though there is no reason to suppose that both types of mechanisms might not be operative simultaneously. In early studies in orally induced hyporesponsiveness in mice, Andre et al.[10] showed that the hyporesponsiveness could be transfered with serum and postulated the suppressive role of immune complexes containing IgA antibody. A number of other investigators, particularly

Table 5
MEDIATORS OF ORAL TOLERANCE

Mediator	Species	Antigen	Assay	Ref.
IgA Ag/Ab	Mice	SRBC	PCA	10
B cell	Mice	Picrylchloride	DTH	12
T cell	Rats	SRBC	PFC	15
	Mice	Ovalbumin	PCA	13
	Mice	Ovalbumin	DTH	20
Serum factor	Mice	SRBC	PFC	14
IgG1	Mice	SRBC	PFC	17
T_s factor	Rats	SRBC	PFC	19
T cell	Mice	Ovalbumin	PA	27
Ly 1^+ T cells	Mice	Bovine serum albumin	PA	104
Ly 2^+ T cells	Mice	Ovalbumin	Antibody	54

those using the SRBC system, showed that the suppression could be transferred with mouse sera but that this activity was attributable to IgG or IgG_1 antibodies and not IgA.[14,17,68] Adoptive transfer studies failed to show that T_s cells were responsible.[14] The factor in the serum was also suppressive for the induction of IgM anti-SRBC responses in normal spleen cultures, and both the in vivo and in vitro suppression was highly specific.[14,68] Characterization of the factor revealed that it was not H-2 restricted and did not block the expression of previously established spleen IgM and anti-SRBC responses. The suppressor factor had a molecular weight of 150,000, was heat stable, and contained Ig determinants but not erythrocyte determinants. Interestingly, IgA and IgE in vitro secondary anti-SRBC responses were not inhibited by the factor.

With oral tolerance to protein antigens, the picture is less clear with regard to serum factors. Thus tolerance to HSA or ovalbumin could not be transferred with sera obtained at 7 to 14 days or 30 to 70 days after stopping feeding.[18,84] However, recently it has been reported that serum taken 4 days after oral immunization with ovalbumin can transfer suppression to syngeneic recipients.[6] Strobel et al.[115] have recently described transfer of tolerance by serum taken 1 hour after ingestion. Activity in serum could be absorbed out with antibody to ovalbumin. Chromatographic analysis revealed these activities to be areas of very low molecular weight, suggesting that the tolerogenic effect was due to low-molecular weight antigens and quickly absorbed breakdown products of ovalbumin. Jackson et al.[116] have demonstrated IgG autoantidiotypic cells to be induced by oral-parenteral immunization with human serum albumin in rabbits. It is possible that such autoantibodies might contribute to oral tolerance, though it should be remembered that previous evidence suggests that rabbits may not respond in the same way as other animal species. However, these findings may offer an explanation for the results of Asherson et al.[12] who showed in mice using picrylchloride that suppression of DTH could be transfered with B cells.

1. Cellular Factors

It is clear that in many of the animal systems discussed that ingestion of antigenic material results in oral tolerance and the production of suppressor cells. These have been demonstrated in Peyer's patches, MLN, and spleens of animals orally tolerized to soluble proteins.[13,16,20,27] These cells have been shown to be of T cell phenotype by using fractionation on nylon wool columns or treatment of cells with anti-thy 1.2.[16,20] These suppressor cells have also been shown to be radiosensitive.[117]

Further evidence for the T cell nature of the suppressor cells is indicated by the fact that pretreatment with cyclophosphamide will abrogate the induction of oral tolerance in the mouse model.[118] However, this has not been found in all models, and Tomasi et

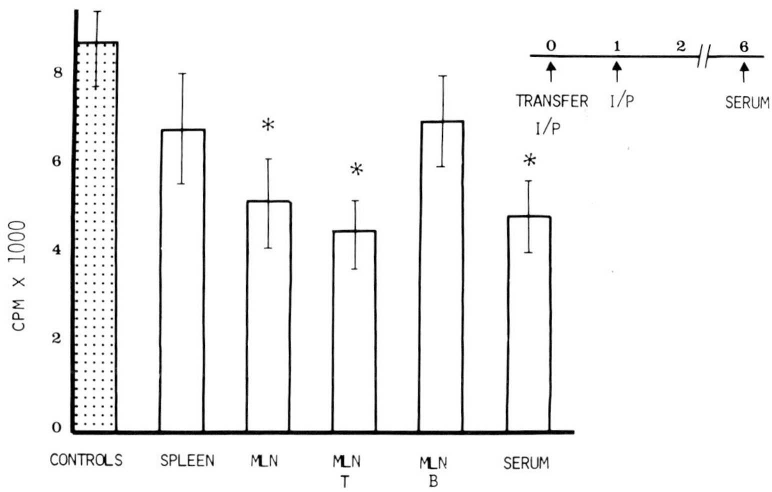

FIGURE 5. Serum IgG antibodies to ovalbumin in recipients of 40 × 10^6 cells from mice immunized with ovalbumin intragastrically. Immunization schedule is as indicated. Cells removed 4 days after intragastric immunization and transferred to syngeneic recipients.

al.[102] report that in their system, the induction of tolerance was unaffected by pretreatment with cyclophosphamide. It has also been suggested that the phenomenon of oral tolerance could be manifested by a functional deletion of T helper (T_h) cells.[88] These authors suggested that small doses of ovalbumin would activate T_s cells and that pretreatment of cyclophosphamide would prevent the development of tolerance but that large dosage resulted in alteration of other T cell functions including diminished carrier-dependent T_h activity.

Recent work with treatment with anti-Ly1 and anti-Ly2 antisera has attempted to elucidate further the phenotype of suppressor cells. Silverman et al.[104] showed that although in vitro antigen-induced proliferation could not be detected in whole lymphocytes preparations from lymph nodes from orally tolerized animals, if cells from these nodes were treated with anti-Ly1 plus complement, then a significant proliferative response was found. This would seem to suggest that T_s cells elicited by oral immuniztion are of the Ly1-positive phenotype. An alternative possibility is that treatment with anti-Ly1 in this mouse system enriches for proliferating Ly2-positive suppressor cells known to be induced by oral immunization[115] and would be part of the contrasuppressor system described for Peyer's patches.[119] This would suggest that failure to observe T_s cell activity in adoptive transfer experiments may be due to the use of whole populations of cells in which suppressor activity is contraregulated.

These findings suggest a complex immunoregulatory network within the Peyer's patches. A commonly suggested view is that oral immunization leads to isotype-specific T_s cells for IgG and IgM which then migrate to systemic lymphoid tissues while T_h cells for IgA remain locally in the intestine.[28] However, these findings would not explain the diminished serum IgA responses found in some studies.[6]

In recent studies with whole bacteria,[54] it has been shown that intragastric immunization with *S. mutans* leads not only to the production of suppressor cells but also to the production of helper cells. Thus both enhancement and suppression can be transferred to syngeneic recipients, and this suggests that what is detected in vivo is the balance between the two systems. With ovalbumin[54] (Figure 5), no helper cells were detected, and this suggests that in the case of soluble protein antigens, the dominant effect is of suppression due to the induction of T_s cells. However, with ovalbumin, tolerance could be transferred with T cells and with serum suggesting that at least two mechanisms were operative simultaneously, though the duration of each is not known (Figure 5).

Characterization of the phenotype of these T cells with antisera revealed that with *S. mutans,* the enhancement could be abolished by treatment with anti-Ly1 antisera, and suppression could be abolished by the pretreatment with anti-Ly2 antisera. In addition, with ovalbumin, suppression could be transferred only by Ly2-positive cells, and no enhancement was seen following the transfer of Ly1-positive cells.[54] It appears therefore that with a complex antigen such as a bacterial cell that both helper and suppressor cells are induced, whereas with a simpler antigen such as ovalbumin, only suppressor cells were induced. However, the inability to detect enhancement may be due either to a lack of helper cells or to inhibited helper cells. An interesting area of current research is into the immunoregulatory networks within the GALT.

Suppressor factors have been described in the rat system with SRBC.[19] These suppressor factors were antigen specific and would act in vitro and in vivo. Thus a number of different mechanisms may be operative according to the animal model and system. It would be interesting for the transfer of oral tolerance to be more fully dissected to determine which mechanisms are necessary for the maintenance of oral tolerance as well as the induction.

V. RELEVANCE OF ANIMAL MODELS TO MAN

It is clear that the use of animal models has allowed major advances in the understanding of the physiology of the gastrointestinal tract. With regard to the secretory system, the use of animal models, particularly those in which genetic and dynamic studies can be performed, has allowed the cellular basis of the secretory system to be examined. The findings have obvious implications with regard to man in terms of vaccination against diseases, particularly of the mucosal surfaces. One of the great difficulties of putting this into practice is the difficulty in prolonging secretory responses, and currently many authors are examining the use of oral adjuvants. There seems to be no doubt that SIgA has the functional capabilities of antigenic exclusion, virus neutralization, inhibition of microbial adherence, and enzyme modulation, but these functions cannot be brought into useful practice unless the secretory response can be stimulated for greater duration than seems likely at present. Understanding the physiology of the gut is an essential prerequisite for the understanding of the pathology of the gut. Animal models have been less useful in the study of certain gut diseases such as celiac disease because of the absence hitherto of suitable models. However, the interesting graft vs. host model of local cell-mediated immunity[73] seems to allow further possibilities of understanding the mechanisms of this and other diseases.

One practical application of the phenomenon or oral tolerance would appear to be in the field of oral desensitization. Although attempts have already been made for desensitization therapy of allergic diseases, these have not been outstandingly successful, and it can be anticipated that with more extensive knowledge about the immunology of the gastrointestinal tract and the systemic manifestations of the immune responses to ingested materials, further attempts will be made in this field. The difficulty in inducing an oral tolerance in primed animals (see above) mitigates against this as an easy option. However, as discussed, a number of studies have shown that tolerance or partial tolerance in primed animals can be achieved, and clearly, this is an area which is worthy of some detailed analysis because of its clinical implications.

In the case of allergy, it is attractive to hypothesize that the dual response to ingested material would have a primary purpose of exclusion of unwanted antigens, allergens, and cross-reacting antigens from the body, and this state would be mediated by the induction of SIgA antibodies. The ingestion of antigen would allow the production of antibodies in most secretions, but antibodies would continue to be secreted only at sites where antigen was still present. Oral tolerance would allow the negation of any damaging systemic reactions to ingested antigens, and this might be particularly pertinent with antigens cross-reacting with host tissue. It may be that the efficient delivery of dimeric IgA from serum into bile via the liver is an extension to this system whereby unwanted antigens and antigen-antibody complexes can be rapidly cleared from the body without any further damaging reactions.

VI. CONCLUSIONS

Deposition of antigenic material in the gut may lead to the simultaneous induction of secretory antibodies and systemic hyporesponsiveness.[27] Under differenct circumstances, such deposition may lead to the simultaneous induction of secretory antibodies and systemic enhancement. This raises intriguing questions as to the relationship between the two systems and also the conditions which determine which of the different types of responses are triggered.

This dual response has hitherto only been demonstrated in the murine model, and it remains to be shown that this is a general phenomenon common to all species. However, this seems likely, since the secretory responses and the systemic hyporesponsiveness have been shown separately in a number of different species.

Immunochemically and functionally the secretory systems of many if not most species appear to be similar. Functional characterization has not been carried out in more than a few species, but many general principles seem to hold. In particular, it seems that secretions in most species can be stimulated locally or centrally and that the gut has a role to play in the general induction of secretory responses. Thus in consideration of secretory responses in the gut itself, both local and general stimulation must be taken into account. With regard to the exciting and relevant area of oral tolerance, there is a remarkable degree of unanimity in the results from all the different animal models. These results suggest that it is a widespread and general phenomenon for systemic hyporesponsiveness to arise after feeding of antigen. This appears at first sight to be difficult to reconcile with the large amount of antigen which is ingested and normally present. Several studies suggest that it is a change in normal antigenic exposure which results in the induction and stimulation of tolerance.

The maintainence of tolerance to ingested antigens is an area of great importance which requires further investigation. It is clear that contrary to the earlier views, antigenic material does get through the stomach and is delivered to the duodenum. This appears to apply to man as well as to other species. The nature of the subsequent systemic immune response depends on the nature of the antigen which has survived, whether it is soluble or particulate, and its molecular size as well as the species of animal, the genetic strains, the dosage of the antigen, and prior antigen exposure. One of the intriguing challenges now that understanding of the oral tolerance system is better is to determine parameters by which previously sensitized individuals may become hyposensitized with antigens. It has great implications in the field of the densensitization of humans along with understanding of the relationship between stimulation of the secretory system and oral tolerance and has widespread potential in veterinary science.

REFERENCES

1. Besredka, A., *Local Immunisation,* Williams & Wilkins, Baltimore, 1927.
2. Davies, A., An investigation into the serological properties of dysentery stools, *Lancet,* 203, 1009, 1922.
3. Cebra, J. J., Kamat, R., Gearhart, P. J., Robertson, S. M., and Tseng, J., The secretory IgA system of the gut, *Ciba Found. Symp.,* 46, 5, 1977.
4. Ogra, P. L. and Karzon, D. T., Distribution of poliovirus antibody in serum, nasopharynx and alimentary tract following segmental immunisation of lower alimentary tract with poliovaccine, *J. Immunol.,* 102, 1423, 1969.
5. Pierce, N. F., The role of antigen form and function in the primary and secondary intestinal immune responses to cholera toxin and toxoid in rats, *J. Exp. Med.,* 148, 195, 1978.
6. Challacombe, S. J., Salivary antibodies and systemic tolerance in mice after oral immunisation with bacterial antigens, *Ann. N.Y. Acad. Sci.,* 409, 177, 1983.
7. Wells, H. G., Studies on the chemistry of anaphylaxis. III. Experiments with isolated proteins, especially those of the hen egg, *J. Infect. Dis.,* 9, 147, 1911.
8. Chase, M. W., Inhibition of experimental drug allergy by prior feeding of the sensitizing agent, *Proc. Soc. Exp. Biol.,* 61, 257, 1946.
9. Tomasi, T. B., Oral tolerance (an overview), *Transplantation,* 29, 353, 1980.
10. André, C., Heremans, J. F., Vaerman, J. P., and Cambiaso, C. L., A mechanism for the induction of immunological tolerance by antigen feeding: antigen-antibody complexes, *J. Exp. Med.,* 142, 1509, 1975.
11. Vaz, N. M., Maia, L. C. S., Hanson, D. G., and Lynch, J. M., Inhibition of homocytotropic antibody responses in adult inbred mice by previous feeding of the specific antigen, *J. Allergy Clin. Immunol.,* 60, 110, 1977.
12. Asherson, G. L., Zembala, M., Perera, M. A. C. C., Mayhew, B., and Thomas, W. R., Production of immunity and unresponsiveness in the mouse by feeding contact sensitizing agents and the role of suppressor cells in the Peyer's patches, mesenteric lymph nodes and other lymphoid tissues, *Cell. Immunol.,* 33, 145, 1977.
13. Ngan, J. and Kind, L. S., Suppressor T cells for IgE and IgG in Peyer's patches of mice made tolerant by the oral administration of ovalbumin, *J. Immunol.,* 120, 861, 1978.
14. Kagnoff, M. F., Effects of antigen feeding on intestinal and systemic immune responses. III. Antigen-specific serum mediated suppression of humoral antibody responses after antigen feeding, *Cell. Immunol.,* 40, 186, 1978.
15. Mattingly, J. A. and Waksman, B. H., Immunologic suppression after oral administration of antigen. I. Specific suppressor cells formed in rat Peyer's patches after oral administration of sheep erythrocytes and their systemic migration, *J. Immunol.,* 121, 1878, 1978.
16. Richman, L. K., Chiller, J. M., Brown, W. R., Hanson, D. G., and Vaz, N. M., Enterically induced immunologic tolerance. I. Induction of suppressor T lymphocytes by intragastric administration of soluble proteins, *J. Immunol.,* 121, 2429, 1978.
17. Chalon, M. P., Milne, R. W., and Vaerman, J. P., *In vitro* immunosuppressive effect of serum of orally immunised mice, *Eur. J. Immunol.,* 9, 747, 1979.
18. Hanson, D. G., Vaz, N. M., Maia, L. C. S., and Lynch, J. M., Inhibition of specific immune responses by feeding protein antigens. III. Evidence against maintenance of tolerance to ovalbumin by orally induced antibodies, *J. Immunol.,* 123, 2337, 1979.
19. Mattingly, J. A. and Waksman, B. H., Immunological suppression after oral administration of antigen. II. Antigen-specific helper and suppressor factors produced by spleen cells of rats fed sheep erythrocytes, *J. Immunol.,* 125, 1044, 1980.
20. Miller, S. D. and Hanson, D. G., Inhibition of specific immune responses by feeding protein antigens. II. Evidence of tolerance and specific active suppression of cell-mediated immune response to ovalbumin, *J. Immunol.,* 123, 2344, 1979.
21. Tomasi, T. B., *The Immune System of Secretions,* Prentice-Hall, Englewood Cliffs, N.J., 1976.
22. Bienenstock, J. and Befus, A. D. M., Mucosal immunology. A review, *Immunology,* 41, 249, 1980.
23. Mestecky, J., McGhee, J. R., Arnold, R. R., Michalek, S. M., Prince, S. M., and Babb, J. C., Selective induction of an immune response in human external secretions by ingestion of bacterial antigen, *J. Clin. Invest.,* 61, 731, 1978.
24. Challacombe, S. J. and Lehner, T., Salivary antibody responses in rhesus monkeys immunised with *Streptococcus mutans* by the oral, submucosal or subcutaneous routes, *Arch. Oral Biol.,* 24, 917, 1980.
25. Swarbrick, E. T., Stokes, C. R., and Soothill, J. F., Absorption of antigens after oral immunisation and the simultaneous induction of specific systemic tolerance, *Gut,* 20, 121, 1979.

26. Walker, W. A., Wu, A. M., and Bloch, K. J., Stimulation by immune complexes of mucus release from goblet cells of the rat small intestine, *Science,* 197, 370, 1977.
27. Challacombe, S. J. and Tomasi, B., Systemic tolerance and secretory immunity after oral immunisation, *J. Exp. Med.,* 152, 1459, 1980.
28. Richman, L. K., Graeff, A. S., Yarchoan, R., and Strober, W., Simultaneous induction of antigen-specific IgA helper T cells and IgG suppressor T cells in the murine Peyer's patch after protein feeding, *J. Immunol.,* 126, 2079, 1981.
29. Challacombe, S. J., Serum and salivary antibodies to *Streptococcus mutans* in relation to the development and treatment of dental caries, *Arch. Oral Biol.,* 25, 495, 1980.
30. Sterzl, J. and Siluerstein, A. M., Development aspects of immunity, *Adv. Immunol.,* 6, 337, 1967.
31. Cooper, M. D. and Lawton, A. R., The development of the immune system, *Sci. Am.,* 2331, 59, 1974.
32. Carter, P. B. and Collins, F. M., Peyers patch responsiveness to salmonella in mice, *J. Reticuloendothelial. Soc.,* 17, 38, 1975.
33. Bienenstock, J., McDermott, M., and Befus, A. D., A common mucosal immune system, in *Immunology of Breast Milk,* Ogra, P. L. and Dayton, D., Eds., Raven Press, New York, 1979, 135.
34. Hanson, D. G. and Morimoto, T., A role of digestion in orally induced tolerance to ovalbumin, *J. Allergy Clin. Immunol.,* 65, 227, 1980.
35. Parrott, D. M. V. and Ferguson, A., Selective migration of lymphocytes within the mouse small intestine, *Immunology,* 26, 571, 1974.
36. Michalek, S. M. McGhee, J. R., and Babb, J. L., Effective immunity to dental caries: dose dependent studies of secretory immunity by oral administration of *Streptococcus mutans* to rats, *Infect. Immun.,* 19, 217, 1977.
37. Vaerman, J. P., Comparative immunobiology of IgA, in *Research in Immunochemistry and Immunobiology,* Kwapinski, J. B., Ed., University Park Press, Baltimore, 1973, 234.
38. Ebersole, J. L., Taubman, M. A., and Smith, D. J., The effect of neonatal thymectomy on the level of salivary and serum immunoglobulins in rats, *Immunology,* 36, 649, 1979.
39. Brandtzaeg, P., Fjellanger, I., and Gjeraldsen, S. J., Human secretory immunoglobulins. I. Salivary secretions from individuals with normal or low levels of serum immunoglobulins, *Scand. J. Haematol. Suppl.,* 12, 1, 1970.
40. Montgomery, P. C., Connell, K. M., Cohn, J., and Skandera, C. A., Remote site stimulation of secretory IgA antibodies following bronchial and gastric stimulation, *Adv. Exp. Med. Biol.,* 107, 113, 1978.
41. Dziaba, K. A., Synkiewicz, Z. M., Binek, M., and Jakubowski, T., The effect of oral immunisation with *E. coli* vaccine on live weight gain in weaned pigs, *Proc. Int. Vet. Soc.,* 165, 121, 1980.
42. Dupont, H. L., Hornick, R. B., and Synder, M. J., Studies of immunity in typhoid fever: protection induced by killed oral vaccines or by primary infection, *Bull. WHO,* 44, 667, 1971.
43. Walker, J., Antibody responses of monkeys to oral and local immunisation with *Streptococcus mutans, Infect. Immun.,* 31, 81, 1981.
44. Linzer, R., Evans, R. T., Emmings, F. G., and Genco, R. J., Use of combined immunisation routes in induction of a salivary immunoglobulin A response to *Streptococcus mutans* in *Macaca fascicularis* monkeys, *Infect. Immun.,* 31, 345, 1981.
45. Taubman, M. A. and Smith, D. J., Effects of local immunisation with glucosyltransferase fractions from *Streptococcus mutans* on dental caries in rats and hamsters, *J. Immunol.,* 118, 710, 1977.
46. Fubara, E. S. and Freter, R., Protection against enteric bacterial infection by secretory IgA antibodies, *J. Immunol.,* 111, 392, 1973.
47. Baljer, G., Hoerstke, M., Dirksen, G., Seitz, A., Sailer, J., and Mayr, A., Vergleichende Untersuchungen uber die Wirksamkeit einer oralen Immunisierung mit hitzeinaktivierten und vermehrungsfahigen avirulenten Gal E- typhimurium-keimen gegen die Salmonellosi des kalbes, *Zentralbl. Veterinaermed.,* 28, 759, 1981.
48. Werner, G. T., and Ulm, K., Evaluation of oral vaccination against mouse typhoid in a new animal model, *Experimentia,* 37, 900, 1981.
49. Newby, T. J., Stokes, C. R., Evans, P. A., and Bourne, F. J., The immune response following oral vaccination with *E. coli, Curr. Top. Vet. Med. Anim. Sci.,* 12, 377, 1981.
50. Sellwood, R., *E. coli* associated porcine neonatal diarrhoea — anti-bacterial activities from colostrum from genetically susceptible and resistant sows, *Infect. Immun.,* 35, 396, 1981.
51. Gillman, R. H., Hornick, R. B., Woodward, W. E., DuPont, M. L., Snyder, M. J., Levine, M. M., and Libonati, J. P., Evaluation of a UDPglucose-4-epimeraseless mutant of *Salmonella typhi* as a live oral vaccine, *J. Infect. Dis.,* 136, 717, 1977.
52. Sutton, R. G. A. and Merson, M. H., Oral typhoid vaccine Ty21a, *Lancet,* i, 523, 1983.
53. Baljer, G., Possibilities and limitations of oral immunisation against *Escherichia coli* in piglets and calves, *Fortschr. Veterinaermed.,* 29, 64, 1979.

54. Challacombe, S. J., Systemic tolerance and salivary antibodies after oral immunisation, *Mucosal Immunity,* Revillard, J. P., Voisin, C., and Wierzbicki, N., Eds., Fondation Franco-Allemande, 1985.
55. Hanson, L. Å., Ahlstedt, S., Andersson, B., Carlsson, B., Cole, M. F., Cruz, J. R., Dahlgren, U., Ericsson, T. H., Jalil, F., Khan, S. R., Mellander, L., Schneerson, R., Svanborg-Eden, C., Soderstrom, T., and Wadsworth, C., Mucosal immunity, *Ann. N.Y. Acad. Sci.,* 409, 1, 1983.
56. Haworth, J. C. and Dilling, L., Concentration of γ-globulin in serum, saliva and nasopharyngeal secretions of infants and children, *J. Lab. Clin. Med.,* 67, 922, 1966.
57. Svennerholm, A. M., Holmgren, J., Hanson, L. Å., Linblad, B. S., Gureshi, F., and Rahimtoola, R. J., Boosting of secretory IgA antibody responses in man by parenteral choleral vaccination, *Scand. J. Immunol.,* 6, 1345, 1977.
58. Pierce, N. F. and Gowans, J. L., Cellular kinetics of the intestinal immune response to cholera toxoid in rats, *J. Exp. Med.,* 142, 1550, 1975.
59. Husband, A. J., An immunisation model for the control of infectious enteritis, *Res. Vet. Sci.,* 25, 173, 1978.
60. Hamilton, S. R., Yardley, J. H., and Brown, G. D., Suppression of local intestinal immunoglobulin A immune response to cholera toxin by subcutaneous administration of cholera toxoid, *Infect. Immun.,* 24, 422, 1979.
61. Beh, K. J., Husband, A. J., and Lascelles, A. K., Intestinal response of sheep to intraperitoneal immunisation, *Immunology,* 37, 385, 1979.
62. Montgomery, P. C., Cohen, C., Skandera, C. A., and Connelly, K. M., Evidence for an IgA anamnestic response in rabbit mammary secretions, in *Immunology of Breast Milk,* Ogra, P. L. and Dayton, D., Eds., Raven Press, New York, 1979, 115.
63. Andrew, E. and Hall, J. G., IgA antibodies in the bile of rats. II. Evidence for immunological memory in secretory immunity, *Immunology,* 45, 177, 1982.
64. Ebersole, J. L. and Molinari, J. A., The induction of salivary antibodies by topical sensitization with particulate and soluble bacterial immunogens, *Immunology,* 34, 969, 1978.
65. Husband, A. M. and Gowans, J. L., The origin and antigen-dependent distribution of IgA containing cells in the intestine, *Cell. Immunol.,* 63, 203, 1981.
66. Singal, D. P., O'Neill, M., Clancy, R., and Bienenstock, J., Functional T cells in rabbit gut mucosal lymphocytes, *Gut,* 17, 235, 1976.
67. Goodacre, R., Davidson, R., Singal, D., and Bienenstock, J., Morphologic and functional characteristics of human intestinal lymphoid cells isolated by a mechanical technique, *Gastroenterology,* 76, 300, 1979.
68. Kagnoff, M. F., Effects of antigen feeding on intestinal and systemic immune responses. II. Similarity between the suppressor factor in mice after erythrocyte-lysate injection and erythrocyte feeding, *Gastroenterology,* 79, 54, 1980.
69. Ferguson, A. and Jarrett, E. E., Hypersensitivity reactions in the small intestine. I. Thymus dependence of experimental 'partial villous atrophy', *Gut,* 16, 114, 1975.
70. Roberts-Thomson, I. C. and Mitchell, G. F., Giardiasis in mice: I. Prolonged infections in certain mouse strains and hypothymic nude mice, *Gastroenterology,* 75, 42, 1978.
71. Rose, M. E. and Long, P. L., Immunity to coccidiosis: interaction *in vitro* between *Eimeria tinnella* and chicken phagocytic cells, in *Biochemistry of Parasite and Host Parasite Relationships,* van de Bossche, H., Ed., Elsevier, Amsterdam, 1976, 449.
72. Ferguson, A., Intraepithelial lymphocytes of the small intestine, *Gut,* 18, 921, 1977.
73. Mowat, A., Tait, R. C., Mackenzie, S., Davies, M. D. J., and Parrott, D. M. V., Analysis of natural effector and suppressor activity by intraepithelial lymphocytes from mouse small intestine, *Clin. Exp. Immunol.,* 52, 191, 1983.
74. MacDonald, T. T. and Ferguson, A., Hypersensitivity reactions in the small intestine. III. The effects of allograft rejection and of graft-versus-host disease on epithelial cell kinetics, *Cell Tissue Kinet.,* 10, 301, 1977.
75. MacDonald, T. T. and Carter, P. B., Cell-mediated immunity to intestinal infection, *Infect. Immun.,* 28, 516, 1980.
76. MacDonald, T. T. and Carter, P. B., Requirement for a bacterial flora before mice generate cells capable of mediating the delayed hypersensitivity reaction to sheep red blood cells, *J. Immunol.,* 122, 2624, 1979.
77. Bellamy, J. E. C. and Nielsen, N. O., Immune-mediated emigration of neutrophils into the lumen of the small intestine, *Infect. Immun.,* 9, 615, 1974.
78. Crabbé, P. A., Nash, D. R., Bazin, H. J., Eyssen, H., and Heremans, J. F., Antibodies of the IgA type in intestinal plasma cells of germ-free mice after oral and parenteral immunisation with ferritin, *J. Exp. Med.,* 130, 723, 1969.
79. Fujita, K. and Finkelstein, R. A., Antitoxic immunity in experimental cholera: comparison of immunity induced perorally and parenterally in mice, *J. Infect. Dis.,* 125, 647, 1972.

80. Pierce, N. F. and Costa, F. T., Priming and suppression of the intestinal immune response to cholera toxoid/toxin by parenteral toxoid in rats, *J. Immunol.*, 124, 307, 1980.
81. Childow, J. W. and Porter, P., The role of oral immunisation in stimulating *Escherichia coli* antibody of the IgM class in porcine colostrum, *Res. Vet. Sci.*, 24, 254, 1978.
82. Stokes, C. R., Newby, T. J., Huntley, J. H., Patel, D., and Bourne, F. J., The immune response of mice to bacterial antigens given by mouth, *Immunology*, 38, 497, 1979.
83. Besredka, A., De l'anaphylaxie. Sixieme memoire de l'anaphylaxie lactique, *Ann. Inst. Pasteur*, 23, 166, 1909.
84. Sewell, H. F., Gell, P. H., and Bazu, M. K., Immune responsiveness and oral immunization, *Int. Arch. Allergy Appl. Immunol.*, 58, 414, 1979.
85. Newby, T. J., Stokes, C. R., Evans, P. A., and Bourne, F. J., The immune response following oral vaccination with *E. coli*, *Curr. Top. Vet. Med. Anim. Sci.*, 12, 377, 1981.
86. Lowney, E. D., Immunological unresponsiveness to a contact sensitizer in man, *J. Invest. Dermatol.*, 51, 411, 1968.
87. Bazin, H. and Platteau, B., Oral feeding of ovalbumin can make rats tolerant to an intraperitoneal injection of dinitrophenylated ovalbumin and *Bordetella pertussis* vaccine, *Biochem. Soc. Trans.*, 5, 1571, 1977.
88. Titus, R. G. and Chiller, J. M., Orally induced tolerance. Definition at the cellular level, *Int. Arch. Allergy Appl. Immunol.*, 65, 323, 1981.
89. Pierce, N. F., Cray, W. C., Jr., and Saccri, J. B., Jr., Oral immunisation against experimental cholera: the role of antigen form and antigen combinations in evoking protection, *Ann. N.Y. Acad. Sci.*, 409, 724, 1983.
90. Kagnoff, M. F., Immunological unresponsiveness after enteric antigen administration, in *Recent Advances in Mucosal Immunity*, Strober, W., Hanson, L., and Sell, K., Eds., Raven Press, New York, 1982, 95.
91. Chiller, J. M., Titus, R. G., and Etlinger, H. M., Cellular dissection of tolerant states induced by the oral route or in neonatal animals, *Dev. Immunol.*, 4, 195, 1979.
92. Kagnoff, M. F., Functional characteristic of Peyer's patch cells. III. Carrier priming of T cells by antigen feeding, *J. Exp. Med.*, 142, 1425, 1975.
93. Asherson, G. L., Perera, M. A. C. C., Thomas, W. R., and Zembala, M., Contact sensitizing agents and the intestinal tract: the production of immunity and unresponsiveness by feeding contact sensitizing agents and the role of suppressor cells, in *Immunology of Breast Milk*, Ogra, P. L. and Dayton, D., Eds., Raven Press, New York, 1979, 19.
94. Mowat, A., Tait, R. C., Mackenzie, S., Davies, M. D. J., and Parrott, D. M. V., Analysis of natural effector and suppressor activity by intraepithelial lymphocytes from mouse small intestine, *Clin. Exp. Immunol.*, 52, 191, 1983.
95. Saklayen, M., Pesce, A. J., Pollak, V. E., and Michael, J. G., Kinetics of oral tolerance: study of variables affecting tolerance induced by oral administration of antigen, *Int. Arch. Allergy Appl. Immunol.*, 73, 5, 1984.
96. Matuhasi, T., Usui, M., and Iwata, M., IgA and IgG enhancing but IgE suppressing characteristics of lipopolysaccharide or cholesterol-ovalbumin conjugate in intubated mice, *Naturwissenschaften*, 69, 397, 1982.
97. Lafont, S., André, C., Andre, F., Gillon, J., and Fargier, M. C., Abrogation by subsequent feeding of antibody response, including IgE, in parenterally immunized mice, *J. Exp. Med.*, 155, 1973, 1982.
98. Bloch, K. J., Perry, R., Bloch, M., and Walker, A., Induction of (partial) systemic tolerance in primed rats subjected to prolonged oral administration of antigen, *Ann. N.Y. Acad. Sci.*, 409, 787, 1983.
99. Michalek, S. M., Kiyono, H., Wannemuehler, M. J., Mosteller, L. M., and McGhee, J. R., Lipopolysaccharide (LPS) regulation of the immune response: LPS influence in oral tolerance induction, *J. Immunol.*, 128, 1992, 1982.
100. Bierme, S. J., Blanc, M., Abral, M., and Fournie, A., Oral Rh treatment for severely immunized mothers, *Lancet*, I, 605, 1979.
101. Sullivan, T. J., Wedner, J. J., and Parker, C. H. W., Densensitization of patients allergic to penicillin using oral penicillin, *J. Allergy Clin. Immunol.*, 65, 195, 1980.
102. Tomasi, T. B., Barr, W. G., Challacombe, S. J., and Curran, G., Oral tolerance and accessory-cell function of Peyer's patches, *Ann. N.Y. Acad. Sci.*, 409, 145, 1983.
103. Korenblat, P. E., Rothberg, R. M., Minden, P., and Farr, R. S., Immune responses of adults after oral and parenteral exposure to bovine serum albumin, *J. Allergy*, 411, 226, 1968.
104. Silverman, G. A., Peri, B. A., and Rothberg, R. M., Systemic antibody responses of different species following ingestion of soluble protein antigens, *Dev. Comp. Immunol.*, 6, 747, 1982.
105. Peri, B. A. and Rothberg, R. M., Circulating antitoxin in rabbits after ingestion of diphtheria toxoid, *Infect. Immun.*, 32, 1148, 1981.

106. Ranges, G. E. and Azar, M. M., Inheritance of tolerance susceptibility to human α globulin in congenic mice, *J. Immunol.*, 123, 1151, 1979.
107. Stokes, C. R., Newby, T. J., and Bourne, F. J., The influence of oral immunisation on local and systemic immune responses to heterologous antigens, *Clin. Exp. Immunol.*, 52, 399, 1983.
108. Bauer, H., Paronetto, F., Burns, W. A., and Einheber, A., The enhancing effect of microbial flora on macrophage function and the immune response, *J. Exp. Med.*, 123, 1013, 1966.
109. McGhee, J. R., Kiyono, H., Michalek, S. M., Babb, J. L., Rosenstreich, D. L., and Mergenhagen, S. E., Lipopolysaccharide regulation of the immune response: T lymphocytes from normal mice suppress mitogenic and immunogenic responses to LPS, *J. Immunol.*, 124, 1603, 1980.
110. Newby, T. J., Stokes, C. R., and Bourne, F. J., Effect of feeding bacterial lipopolysaccharide and dextran sulphate on the development of oral tolerance to contact sensitising agents, *Immunology*, 41, 617, 1980.
111. Saklayen, M., Pesce, A. J., Pollak, V. E., and Michael, J. G., Induction of oral tolerance in mice unresponsive to bacterial lipopolysaccharide, *Infect. Immun.*, 41, 1383, 1983.
112. Krco, C. J., Challacombe, S. J., Lafuse, W. P., David, C. S., and Tomasi, T. B., Jr., Expression of Ia antigens by mouse Peyer's patch cells, *Cell. Immunol.*, 57, 420, 1981.
113. Richman, L. K., Graeff, A. S., and Strober, W., Antigen presentation by macrophage enriched cells from the mouse Peyer's patch, *Cell. Immunol.*, 62, 110, 1981.
114. Mayrhofer, G., Physiology of the intestinal immune system. in *Local Immune Responses in the Gut*, Newby, T. J. and Stokes, C. R., CRC Press, Boca Raton, Fla., 1984, chap. 1.
115. Strobel, S., Mowat, A. M., Drummond, H. E., Pickening, M. G., and Ferguson, A., Immunological responses to fed protein antigens in mice. II. Oral tolerance for CMI is due to activation of cyclophosphamide sensitive cells by gut processed antigen, *Immunology*, 49, 451, 1983.
116. Jackson, D. E., Lally, E. T., Nakamura, M. C., and Montgomery, P. C., Migration of IgA-bearing lymphocytes into salivary glands, *Cell. Immunol.*, 63, 203, 1981.
117. Hanson, D. G., Vaz, N. M., Rawlings, L. A., and Lynch, J. M., Inhibition of specific immune responses by feeding protein antigens. II. Effects of prior passive and active immunization, *J. Immunol.*, 122, 2261, 1979.
118. Mowat, A. M., Strobel, S., Drummond, H. E., and Ferguson, A., Immunological responses to fed protein antigens in mice. I. Reversal of oral tolerance to ovalbumin by cyclophosphamide, *Immunology*, 45, 105, 1982.
119. Green, D. R. and St. Martin, S., Suppression and contrasuppression in the regulation of gut-associated immune responses, *Ann. N.Y. Acad. Sci.*, 409, 284, 1983.

Index

INDEX

A

Acetylsalicylic acid (ASA; aspirin), 26, 89—90, 93
Addison's disease, 27—28, 30
Additives, food, 85—95
Adjuvants, oral, 118
Adoptive transfer, 7, 10, 116
Age, effect of, 27, 29, 32, 106—107
Alcohol, 26, 71
Allergens, 12—13, 32—33, 50, 88
Allergy and food intolerance, 69—81
 in adults, 75—79
 in children, 70—75
 clinical patterns, 70—71
 methods of diagnosis, 79—81
Amaranth, 88, 90, 93
Anaphylaxis, 77, 111
Anemia, 27—31, 46, 51, 71, 77
Angioedema, 73, 75, 92
Animal models, 100—119
Ankylosing spondylitis, 95
Annatto, 89, 92—93
Antibody-dependent cell-mediated cytotoxicity, 3—4, 13, 15, 48, 50
Antigen exclusion, 101
Antigen-presenting cells, 155
Antigens
 bacterial, 110, 112
 insoluble, 109
 particulate, 103, 105
 prior exposure to, effect of, 107—108, 113—114
 soluble, 105, 109, 117
 T-cell dependent, 112, 114
 thymus-independent, 112
Anti-inflammatory agents, 26, 32
Antioxidants, 86, 89, 91—92
Antireticulin antibody, 35, 70
Arachidonic acid metabolites, 88
Arthritis, 49, 51, 70, 77
Arthus reaction, 38
Ascaris, 11, 14
Aspirin, 26, 86—90, 93
Asthma, 72, 74—75, 86—91, 93
Autoantibodies, 28, 30, 49
Autoantidiotypic cells, 116
Autoimmune diseases, 27—28, 30, 39, 51

B

Bacteria, 3, 77, 105, 110, 112, 117—118
Basophils, 4, 8, 12, 34
B cell antigen, 39—40
B-cell generating factor, 13
B cells, 8, 31, 46, 51
Benzoates, 86, 89—94
Benzoic acid, 73, 89
Bixin, 89—90
Boosting, oral, 107
Bowel disease, inflammatory, see also Irritable bowel syndrome, 38, 45—55
Butylated hydroxyanisole (BHA), 91—92
Butylated hydroxytoluene (BHT), 91—92

C

Caffeine, 78
Campylobacter pyloridis, 32
Carotenoid extracts, 89
Carrageenan, 94
Celiac disease, 26, 34—42, 44—45, 55, 72
Cell-mediated immunity, 108
 celiac disease, 36—39
 gastritis, 29—31
 inflammatory bowel disease, 45—46, 49—53
Challenge tests, 73—74, 77—80
Cholera toxin, 107, 109, 112
Chromates, 94
Cinnamate, 91
Coccidia, 5, 9—10
Coccidiosis, 4—6
Colitis
 infantile, 41
 milk-induced, 72
 ulcerative, 26, 41, 45—49, 51—55
Complement, 31, 34, 49, 54
Contrasuppressor system, 117
Cow's milk protein intolerance, 26, 40—44, 55, 72
Crohn's disease, 26, 35, 41, 45—51, 53—55
Cromoglycate, 33—34, 49
Cyclooxygenase pathway, 87—88
Cyclophosphamide, 116—117
Cytotoxic tests, 80

D

Dermatitis
 atopic, 73—74, 86
 contact, 94
 herpetiformis, 27, 72
Densensitization therapy, 118
Diabetes mellitus, insulin-dependent, 27—28, 30
Diets
 diagnostic, 79—80
 elimination, 34, 74—75, 79—80, 87
 gluten-free, 34, 36—37, 44—45
 milk-free, 54
Digestion, inborn errors of, 70—72
Duodenitis, 45
Dyes, 86—90, 92—93

E

Echinococcus, 6

Eczema, 72, 74—75, 94
Eimeria, 5, 9
Endotoxin, 51
Entamoeba histolytica, 4
Enzyme deficiencies, 70—71, 76—78
Eosinophil chemotactic factor of anaphylaxis (ECF-A), 34
Eosinophils, 4, 7, 11, 14—15, 33—34
Epilepsy, 74—75
Erythrosine, 89, 92
Escherichia coli, 49, 52—53, 105
Expulsion, worm, 7—9, 14

F

Fasciola, 6
Flora, normal bacterial, 108, 115
Flukes, 6
Food colors and additives, 73, 78, 85—95
Food intolerance and allergy, 86, 92—93
  in adults, 75—79
  in children, 70—75
  clinical patterns, 70—71
  in Crohn's disease, 50
  in eczema, 74
  foods commonly involved in, 75—76, 79
  frequency of, 92—93
  in gastritis, 32—33
  in infantile colitis, 41
  methods of diagnosis, 79—81
  susceptibility to, 114
Food aversion, 70
Food intolerance, 70—72, 74—80, 86, 92—93
Food residues, fermentation of, 70, 77
Food storage and processing, changes with, 78—79
Food toxicity, 77—78

G

Gas, intestinal, 77
Gastritis, 26—34, 55
Gastroenteritis, eosinophilic, 76
Genetic factors, 94—95, 112, 114—115
Genetic studies, 14, 16, 28, 38, 55
Giardia lamblia, 4
Giardia muris, 4—5
Giardiasis, 4—5, 11, 41
Gliadin, 34—37, 55
γ-Globulin, human (HGG), 111, 114
Gluten, 26, 34—40, 55, 70, 72, 94
Goblet cells, 4, 6, 8
Graft vs. host disease, 37, 108
Granulocytes, 6
Granulomata, 48—50, 52
Gut-associated lymphoid tissue (GALT), 101
  chronic GI diseases, 55
  mucosal immune responses, 103, 106
  parasite infections, 3—4, 6—7
  systemic immune responses, 115, 118

H

Haemonchus contortus, 10—11
Hayfever, 86
Helminths, 2, 4, 12—15
Heterophils, 10
Histamine, 33, 78—79, 86—88, 93
HLA system, 38—40, 43, 94—95
Hookworms, 9, 12, 14
5-Hydroxyeicosatetraenoic acid (5HETE), 34
Hymenolepis nana, 15
Hyperactivity, 75, 87
Hypergammaglobulinemia, 9
Hyperresponsiveness, immune, abnormal, 46, 55
Hypersensitivity
  delayed type (DTH), 94, 108, 111—115
    celiac disease, 37—38
    gastritis, 31
    inflammatory bowel disease, 46
    parasitic infection, 4
  to food, 86
  immediate, 8, 10, 12—13, 33, 36, 88
  type I, 42, 93
  type III, 42—44
  type IV, 43
Hyperventilation syndrome, 81
Hypogammaglobulinemia, 11, 46, 55
Hypolactasia, 40, 71
Hypoparathyroidism, 27—28
Hyporesponsiveness, 101, 109—111

I

IgA antibodies
  anti-parasite, 5, 7, 10—11
  in local immunity, 100, 102—103, 113
  in milk sensitivity, 42
  in pernicious anemia, 29
IgD antibodies, 94
IgE antibodies
  in food allergy, 70, 74, 76, 93
  in gastrointestinal diseases, 32, 34
IgG antibodies, 5, 9—10, 29, 43—44
Immune complexes, circulating, 35—36, 42, 47, 49, 52—54, 119
Immune exclusion, 101—102, 115
Immunization, 101—114
Immunodeficiency, 36, 55
Immunoglobulin A (IgA)
  in celiac disease, 35
  deficiency of, 42—43, 46, 55
  in responses to intestinal parasites, 5, 7—11, 15
  secretory (SIgA), 3, 29, 42, 106—107, 119
Immunoglobulin E (IgE), 3, 8, 12—13, 15, 33—34
Immunoglobulin G (IgG), 3, 5, 7, 15, 102
Immunoglobulin M (IgM), 35, 47
Immunosuppression, 9, 15—16
Infections, intestinal, 2

Inflammatory reactions, 5—8, 10, 13—14
Inflammatory bowel disease, 45—55
Intrinsic factor antibody, 28—32
Irritable bowel syndrome, 75, 79
Isotype switching, 4

J

Joint pains, 77

K

Killer (K) cells, 48, 108

L

β-Lactoglobulin, 42
Lactose intolerance, 40—41, 54
Lectins, 40, 55, 79
Leukocytes, 11
Leukotrienes, 34
Lipopolysaccharide (LPS), 49, 52, 112, 115
Lupus erythematosis, 51
Lymphoblasts, 5, 10, 43

M

Macrophage migration inhibition factor, 37, 39
Macrophages, 5, 10, 48—49, 52, 115
Malnutrition, 46
Mast cells
  in antiparasitic responses, 6—7, 11—12
  in aspirin analgesia, 87
  in gastrointestinal diseases, 33—34, 49
  mucosal (MMC), 4, 12—14, 36
Mastomys natalensis, 33
Memory, immunological, 107—108
Metabolism, disorders of, 71—72
Migraine, 74—75, 77
Milk, breast, 41
Milk sensitivity, 54, 92
Mucosa, jejunal, 37
Myasthenia gravis, 27—28
Myxedema, 27

N

Natural killer (NK) cells, 4, 48, 108
Nematodes, 7—13
Nematospiroides dubius, 5, 9, 14—16
Neutrophils, 7, 44, 48—49, 52, 108
Nickel, 94
Nippostrongylus brasiliensis, 8—9, 13—15, 37
Norbixin, 89—90

O

Oesophagostomatum columbianum, 11
Oral tolerance, 16, 101—102, 106—119
Ostertagia circumcincta, 10—11
Ovalbumin, 105—106, 111—114, 117—118

P

Panhypogammaglobulinemia, 30—31
Paprika, 89
Parasites, intestinal, 1—16, 108
  in domestic animals, 9—11
  immune effector mechanisms, 3—4
  immunity, 2—3
  immunological consequences, 12—16
  in laboratory models, 4—9
  in man, 11—12
Parietal cell antibody, 29—32
Pathophysiological changes, 4, 7
Penicillins, 33
Peptic ulcer disease, 32
Peru balsam, 92
Peyer's patches, 102—103, 108, 111—112, 115—117
Platyhelminths, 6—7, 13
Ponceau 4R, 88, 90, 92
Priming, 107, 110, 113
Proctitis, hemorrhagic, 76
Prostaglandin synthesis, 87—88
Protein intolerance, 71
Protein-tartrazine conjugates, 94
Protozoa, 2, 4—6
Pseudoallergic reactions, 78
Pulse test, 80

R

Rat mast cell protease (RMCP II), 8, 13—14
Rhinitis, 72, 74, 86—87, 93
Rinkel technique, 80
Roundworms, 11

S

Saffron, 89
Salicylates, 87—88, 90
Saliva, 101—108
Salmonella typhimurium, 105, 107
Schistosoma mansonii, 34
Scromboid poisoning, 78—79
Secretory component (SC), 103
Secretory responses, 103—108
Self-cure, 7, 10
Sensitization, 50, 75, 91, 113
Shigella, 105
Sicca syndrome, 27

Skin testing, 37—38, 51
Slow-reacting substance of anaphylaxis (SRS-A), 88
Smoking, 51, 54
Soya protein enteropathy, 26, 43—45, 55, 72
Sporozoites, 10
Staphylococcus aureus, 49
Steroids, 34
Streptococcal antigen I/II, 109—111
Streptococcus mutans, 102—108, 110, 112, 114, 117—118
Strongyloides stercoaalis, 12
Sunset yellow, 73, 88, 90, 92—93

T

Taenia taeniaformis, 6
Tapeworms, 6
Tartrazine, 73, 86—89, 92—94
T cells
  in Crohn's disease, 46—47, 49
  helper, 31, 39, 47, 53, 94, 102, 114, 116—118
  in pernicious anemia, 31
  in responses to intestinal parasites, 3—4, 6—9
  suppressor, 31, 39, 47, 53, 94, 102, 114, 116—118
  in ulcerative colitis, 51—52
Thyroiditis, Hashimoto's, 27—28
Thyrotoxicosis, 27
Tobacco, 26
Tolerance, systemic, to antigens, 15—16
Trichinella spiralis, 7—9, 13—15
Trichostrongylus colubriformis, 8, 10, 14
Trichostrongylus vitrinus, 11
Trichuris, 12
Tyramine, 78—79

U

Ulcerative colitis, 26, 41, 45—49, 51—55
Urticaria, 73—75, 78, 86—87, 89—93

V

Vaccines, 105
Vanillin, 91
Vibrio cholerae, 105, 107
Viruses, 53—54
Vitamin B_{12}, 28—30
Vitiligo, 27

Z

Zinc deficiency, 46